NSNA Review Series

Fluids and Electrolytes

Consulting Editor
Margaret A. McEntee, Ph.D., R.N., M.S., B.S.N.
Assistant Professor
University of Maryland School of Nursing
Baltimore, Maryland

Reviewer
Grace M. Gil, R.N., M.S.N., B.S.N.
Instructor
Central Florida Community College
Ocala, Florida

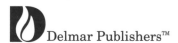
Delmar Publishers™

I(T)P An International Thomson Publishing Company

Albany • Bonn • Boston • Cincinnati • Detroit • London • Madrid • Melbourne
Mexico City • New York • Pacific Grove • Paris • San Francisco • Singapore • Tokyo
Toronto • Washington

Developed for Delmar Publishers Inc. by Visual Education Corporation, Princeton, New Jersey.
Sponsoring Editor: Patricia Casey
Project Director: Theresa C. Moore
Production Supervisor: Christine Osborne
Proofreading Management: Emily R. Jacoby
Electronic Preparation: Cynthia C. Feldner
Electronic Production: Elise Dodeles, Lisa Evans-Skopas
Cover Designer: Paul C. Uhl, DESIGNASSOCIATES
Text Designer: Circa 86

Copyright © 1997

By Delmar Publishers
a division of International Thomson Publishing Inc.

The ITP logo is a trademark under license.

Printed in the United States of America

For more information contact:

Delmar Publishers
3 Columbia Circle, Box 15015
Albany, New York 12212-5015

International Thomson Publishing
Europe
Berkshire House 168-173
High Holborn
London, WCIV 7AA
England

Thomas Nelson Australia
102 Dodds Street
South Melbourne, 3205, Victoria
Australia

Nelson Canada
1120 Birchmont Road
Scarborough, Ontario, M1K 5G4
Canada

International Thomson Editores
Campos Eliscos 385, Piso 7
Col Polanco
11560 Mexico, D.F.
Mexico

International Thomson Publishing GmbH
Konigswinterer strasse 418
53227 Bonn, Germany

International Thomson Publishing Asia
#05-10 Henderson Building
221 Henderson Road
Singapore 0315

International Thomson Publishing Japan
Hirakawacho Kyowa Building, 3F
2-2-1 Hirakawa-cho
Chiyoda-ku, Tokyo 102
Japan

1 2 3 4 5 6 7 8 9 10 XXX 03 02 01 00 99 98 97 96

Library of Congress Cataloging–in–Publication Data

Fluids and electrolytes / consulting editor, Margaret A. McEntee ;
    reviewer, Grace M. Gil.
        p.   cm. — (NSNA review series)
    Includes bibliographical references.
    ISBN: 0-8273-7641-3
    1. Water-electrolyte imbalances—Nursing—Outlines, syllabi, etc. 2. Water-electrolyte imbalances—
Nursing—Examinations, questions, etc. 3. Body fluid disorders—Nursing—Outlines, syllabi, etc. 4. Body fluid
disorders—Nursing—Examinations, questions, etc. I. McEntee, Margaret Aurelia. II. Gil, Grace M. III. Series.
    [DNLM: 1. Nursing Care—methods—outlines. 2. Nursing Care—methods—examination questions.
3. Water-Electrolyte Imbalance—nursing—examination questions. 4. Fluid Therapy—nursing—outlines.
5. Fluid Therapy—nursing—examination questions. WY 18.2 F646 1997]
RC630.F5925   1997
616.3'9—dc20
DNLM/DLC
for Library of Congress   96–24184
                                                                                                      CIP

Titles in Series

Maternal-Newborn Nursing

Pediatric Nursing

Nursing Pharmacology

Medical-Surgical Nursing

Psychiatric Nursing

Gerontologic Nursing

Health Assessment and Physical Examination

Nutrition and Diet Therapy

Community Health Nursing

Fluids and Electrolytes

Critical Care Nursing

Series Advisory Board

Series Review Board

Contents

Notice to the Reader

Publisher does not warrant or guarantee any of the products described herein or perform any independent analysis in connection with any of the product information contained herein. Publisher does not assume, and expressly disclaims, any obligation to obtain and include information other than that provided for it by the manufacturer.

The reader is expressly warned to consider and adopt all safety precautions that might be indicated by the activities herein and to avoid all potential hazards. By following the instructions contained herein, the reader willingly assumes all risks in connection with such instructions.

The publisher makes no representation or warranties of any kind, including, but not limited to, warranties of fitness for a particular purpose or for merchantability; neither are any such representations implied with respect to the material set forth herein, and the publisher takes no responsibility with respect to such material. The publisher shall not be liable for any special, consequential, or exemplary damages resulting, in whole or part, from a reader's use of, or reliance upon, this material.

Preface

The NSNA Review Series is a multiple-volume series designed to help nursing students review course content and prepare for course tests.

Chapter elements include:

Overview—lists the main topic headings for the chapter

Nursing Highlights—gives significant nursing care concepts relevant to the chapter

Glossary—features key terms used in the chapter that are not defined within the chapter

Enhanced Outline—consists of short, concise phrases, clauses, and sentences that summarize the main topics of course content; focuses on nursing care and the nursing process; includes the following elements:
- *Client Teaching Checklists:* shaded boxes that feature important issues to discuss with clients; designed to help students prepare client education sections of nursing care plans
- *Nurse Alerts:* shaded boxes that provide information that is of critical importance to the nurse, such as danger signs or emergency measures connected with a specific condition or situation
- *Locators:* finding aids placed across the top of the page that indicate the main outline section being covered on a particular 2-page spread within the context of other main section heads
- *Textbook reference aids:* boxes labeled "See text pages ____," which appear in the margin next to each main head, to be used by students to list the page numbers in their textbook that cover the material presented in that section of the outline
- *Cross-references:* references to other parts of the outline, which identify the relevant section of the outline by using the numbered and lettered outline levels (e.g., "same as section I,A,1,b" or "see section II,B,3")

Chapter Tests—review and reinforce chapter material through questions in a format similar to that of the National Council Licensure Examination for Registered Nurses (NCLEX-RN); answers follow the questions and contain rationales for both correct and incorrect answers

Comprehensive Test—appears at the end of the book and includes items that review material from each chapter

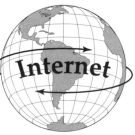

1

Introduction

NURSING HIGHLIGHTS

1. Electrolyte and fluid imbalances are commonly associated with disease states or injury; they rarely occur alone.
2. The nurse should be aware that, for clients who are elderly or obese, total body fluids account for a lesser percentage of body weight; such clients can become dehydrated more rapidly than younger or leaner clients.
3. Infants need more fluids per kg of body weight than do adults; because infant kidneys do not concentrate urine well, dehydration can occur rapidly.
4. The nurse should monitor changes in baseline vital signs and laboratory test results that indicate fluid and electrolyte imbalances; such imbalances can develop rapidly, sometimes as the result of medical interventions.

GLOSSARY

colloid—a substance such as a protein that, when dissolved or dispersed in a liquid, diffuses through a membrane either very slowly or not at all
edema—a perceptible accumulation of interstitial fluid

homeostasis—the state of equilibrium of the internal environment

hormone—a chemical substance formed in one organ or gland and carried in the blood to another organ or part of the body that it stimulates to functional activity

plasma—intravascular fluid consisting of water, ions, and colloidal material (i.e., blood minus blood cells)

serum—the fluid portion of the blood obtained after coagulation; often used interchangeably with the term *plasma* in clinical settings, but technically it is plasma without fibrinogen

ENHANCED OUTLINE

See text pages
_____

I. Basic concepts: Complex structures and functions in the human body at the level of molecules, cells, tissues, organs, and organ systems require water; fluids constitute 60% of adult body weight.

A. Fluid compartments: not discrete sacs, but areas in the body where water and electrolytes are found
  1. Intracellular: fluid existing inside the cell; accounts for 40% of body weight in healthy adults
  2. Extracellular: fluid existing outside the cell, found in tissue spaces and blood vessels; accounts for 20% of body weight in healthy adults
    a) Intravascular: fluid found in the blood vessels (e.g., veins, arteries, capillaries); accounts for 5% of body weight in healthy adults
    b) Interstitial: fluid found between cells in tissue spaces (e.g., spaces between cells of skeletal muscle); accounts for 15% of body weight in healthy adults
  3. Variations in amount of body fluids
    a) Newborns have higher total body fluids than adults (70%–80% of body weight).
    b) The elderly have lower total body fluids than younger adults (46%–52% of body weight).
    c) Obese clients have lower total body fluids than lean clients of the same age and sex, because fat cells contain little water.
    d) Women have lower total body fluids than men of the same age and weight, because women have a higher proportion of fat.
  4. Variations in distribution of body fluids
    a) In newborns, more than half of the fluid (70%–80% of body weight) is found in the extracellular fluid (ECF) compartment; because ECF is lost more readily than intracellular fluid (ICF), newborns are highly susceptible to dehydration.

b) During infancy, distribution shifts; by age 1, ECF accounts for 30% of body weight, and ICF for 34%; by age 2, ECF constitutes 24% of body weight, and ICF 40%.

c) By puberty, the adult fluid distribution is reached; ECF constitutes 20% of body weight, and ICF 40%.

B. Fluid functions: Water is essential for cellular metabolism; a 20% fluid loss is fatal.

1. Transport of nutrients (e.g., glucose), electrolytes (e.g., sodium, potassium), and oxygen to cells: Exchange of nutrients occurs in the capillary bed.

2. Transport of wastes (e.g., urea, carbon dioxide) from cells: Removal of wastes occurs in the capillary bed.

3. Regulation of body temperature: Body temperature is mildly elevated in clients with water deficit (dehydration, hypernatremia), possibly related to lack of available fluid for sweating.

4. Lubrication of joints and membranes

5. Medium in which chemical reactions occur

C. Fluid constituents: water, electrolytes, proteins, organic acids, nutrients, waste products, gases

1. Electrolytes: substances that dissolve in water into electrically charged particles called ions

   a) Charges carried by electrolytes

      (1) Cations: positively charged ions (e.g., sodium [Na^+], calcium [Ca^{++}], potassium [K^+], magnesium [Mg^{++}])

      (2) Anions: negatively charged ions (e.g., chloride [Cl^-], bicarbonate [HCO_3^-], phosphate [HPO_4^{--}], sulfate [SO_4^{--}])

   b) Measurement of electrolyte activity

      (1) Milliequivalents per liter (mEq/L): measure of the number of anions or cations available to combine with other anions or cations in a solution

         (a) Most commonly used measure of electrolyte activity in clinical settings in United States is mEq.

         (b) To calculate mEq, divide the milligram-equivalent weight (atomic number divided by 1000) of the ion by its valence, or combining power (e.g., milligram-equivalent weight of Na^+ = 23[atomic weight]/1000 = 23 mg; 1 mEq Na^+ = 23 mg/1[valence] = 23 mg).

         (c) One mEq of cation will always react with one mEq of anion.

      (2) Milligrams per deciliter (mg/dl): measure of the weight of a substance dissolved in 100 ml (1 dl) of water

      (3) Millimoles per liter (mmol/L): measure of the milligram-equivalent weight of a substance dissolved in 1 liter of water

         (a) Countries using the Système Internationale favor this measure for expressing body fluid content.

         (b) To convert mmol/L, use mEq/L = mmol/L × valence of the electrolyte (e.g., 1 mmol Na^+ × 1[valence] = 1 mEq Na^+; 1 mmol Ca^{++} × 2[valence] = 2 mEq Ca^{++}).

c) Normal electrolyte constituents of ICF: Within a compartment, anions and cations are present in equal numbers.
   (1) Cations: positive charge
       (a) K^+: major cation of ICF, 141–150 mEq/L; much higher than in ECF
       (b) Mg^{++}: 27 mEq/L
       (c) Na^+: 10 mEq/L
       (d) Ca^{++}: 2 mEq/L
   (2) Anions: negative charge
       (a) HPO_4^{--}: major anion of ICF, 100 mEq/L
       (b) HCO_3^-: 10 mEq/L
       (c) Cl^-: 1 mEq/L
d) Normal electrolyte constituents of ECF: values commonly obtained in clinical setting to assess electrolyte balance (plasma electrolytes)
   (1) Cations: positive charge
       (a) Na^+: major electrolyte of ECF, 142 mEq/L; much higher than in ICF

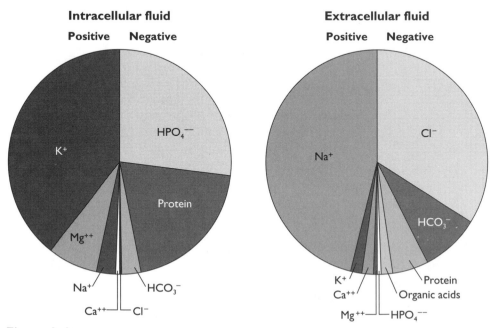

Figure 1–1
Proportions of Charged Particles in Body Fluids

      (b) K^+: 5 mEq/L

      (c) Ca^{++}: 5 mEq/L

      (d) Mg^{++}: 2 mEq/L

   (2) Anions: negative charge

      (a) Cl^-: major anion of ECF, 104 mEq/L

      (b) HCO_3^-: 27 mEq/L

      (c) HPO_4^{--}: 2 mEq/L

2. Proteins: nitrogen-based compounds that are essential to all living organisms; carry a negative charge and play a role in maintaining the charge neutrality of each fluid compartment; blood proteins diffuse little or not at all across membranes

  a) Plasma proteins: albumin, globulin, and fibrinogen (a clotting agent)

  b) Serum proteins: albumin and globulin

   (1) Serum albumin: main blood protein; constitutes about 50% of total protein in intracellular fluid; main function is to maintain plasma colloidal osmotic pressure

   (2) Serum globulin: assists in maintaining plasma colloidal osmotic pressure (See section II,E of this chapter for an explanation of the role of colloidal osmotic [oncotic] pressure in fluid movement in the capillary bed.)

3. Organic acids: carbon-based compounds that carry a negative charge and play a role in maintaining the charge neutrality of each fluid compartment

4. Nutrients, waste products, and gases: Transported by body fluids, these components do not play a significant role in maintaining charge neutrality, but may affect various aspects of fluid and electrolyte balance in specific circumstances addressed in later chapters.

II. Fluid movement in the body: Fluids move constantly and rapidly between compartments to maintain homeostasis.

See text pages

A. Definitions

  1. Solution: incorporation of a solid, liquid, or gas into a fluid that results in a uniform (homogenous) liquid

  2. Solute: substance (e.g., solid, liquid, gas) dissolved in a solution

  3. Solvent: liquid that holds a solute in solution

  4. Membrane: thin layer of tissue that serves as the covering of an organ or divides a space

  5. Permeability: capacity of a membrane to allow fluids and other substances (e.g., ions, proteins) to pass through it

    a) Selectively permeable membrane: refers to a living membrane that allows some substances to pass through freely while blocking others

    b) Semipermeable membrane: refers to an artificial membrane that allows some substances to pass through freely while blocking others

  6. Pressure gradient: difference in pressure (osmotic or hydrostatic) that causes fluids to flow

    a) Osmotic pressure: pressure that develops when two solutions with different solute concentrations are separated by a membrane permeable to the solvent, resulting in a flow of solvent across the membrane (See section II,C of this chapter for a discussion of osmosis.)

    b) Hydrostatic pressure: force of fluid pressing outward against a membrane when a fluid is at equilibrium (See section II,D of this chapter for a discussion of hydrostatic pressure related to filtration.)

B. Diffusion: process by which a solute (e.g., gas, ion) moves in all directions through a solution
    1. Net movement from an area of greater solute concentration to an area of lesser solute concentration
    2. Occurs between fluid compartments if membrane is permeable to solute (e.g., Oxygen diffuses from capillary bed into cells.)
    3. No energy expended by cell

C. Osmosis: movement of a solvent (e.g., water) across a solute-impermeable membrane from an area of lesser concentration (less solute) to an area of greater concentration (more solute); osmotic pressure draws or pulls solvent across a membrane; occurs without expending cellular energy
    1. Osmolality (tonicity): number of osmotically active particles dissolved in 1 kg of water
        a) Osmols (Osm) and milliosmols (mOsm) measure the osmotic pressure (osmotic pull) exerted by particles in a solution.
        b) Serum osmolality is used to monitor electrolytes in the intravascular fluid in clinical settings (normal range 280–295 mOsm/kg).
    2. Iso-osmolar (isotonic): containing approximately the same solute concentration as plasma; normal osmolality range for IV solutions is 240–340 mOsm/kg; plasma osmolality probably not disturbed over this range because of dilution factor presented by total plasma volume
        a) Examples: isotonic or normal saline (0.9% sodium chloride [NaCl]), 310 mOsm; lactated Ringer's, 275 mOsm
        b) Activity: no net movement of solvent when two solutions are iso-osmolar
    3. Hyperosmolar (hypertonic): containing a higher solute concentration than the upper end of the normal osmolality range for IV solutions (greater than 340 mOsm/kg); having a solute concentration sufficiently higher than plasma to disturb plasma osmolality
        a) Example: 3% NaCl (hyperosmolar saline), 1025 mOsm
        b) Activity: Hyperosmolar solutions exert greater osmotic pressure (osmotic pull); blood cells in hyperosmolar solutions shrink as water moves out of the cells.
    4. Hypo-osmolar (hypotonic): containing a lower solute concentration than the lower end of the normal osmolality range for IV solutions

(less than 240 mOsm/kg); having a solute concentration sufficiently lower than plasma to disturb plasma osmolality
   a) Example: 0.45% NaCl (hypo-osmolar saline), 155 mOsm
   b) Activity: Hypo-osmolar solutions exert less osmotic pressure; blood cells in hypo-osmolar solutions swell as water moves into the cells.

D. Filtration: transfer of fluid across a selectively permeable membrane from a region of high pressure to a region of low pressure; driving force is hydrostatic pressure, which pushes fluid across a membrane

E. Movement of fluids in the capillary bed: Movement of fluids out of the capillaries (intravascular space), into interstitial space (tissue space, or space between the cells of a tissue), and then back into capillaries allows nutrient delivery and waste product removal at the cellular level.
   1. Definitions
      a) Plasma colloidal osmotic (oncotic) pressure: osmotic pressure exerted by nondiffusible proteins (colloids) in plasma (e.g., albumin, globulin)
      b) Tissue colloidal osmotic (oncotic) pressure: osmotic pressure exerted by nondiffusible proteins (colloids) in interstitial fluid
   2. Forces acting at the arterial end of the capillary bed
      a) The plasma hydrostatic pressure is higher than the tissue hydrostatic pressure.
      b) The plasma colloidal osmotic (oncotic) pressure is higher than the tissue colloidal osmotic (oncotic) pressure.
      c) The plasma hydrostatic pressure is higher than the plasma colloidal pressure.
      d) Net force pushes water and electrolytes out of capillaries into interstitial space.
   3. Forces acting at the venous end of the capillary bed
      a) The plasma hydrostatic pressure is lower than the tissue hydrostatic pressure, because fluids have moved out of the capillaries.
      b) The plasma colloidal osmotic pressure remains higher than tissue colloidal osmotic pressure, because proteins that produce it are unable to diffuse across the capillary membranes.
      c) Net force pulls fluid from interstitial space into capillaries.
   4. 90% of filtered fluid is resorbed in the capillary bed; 10% is returned by the lymphatic system.

F. Active transport: movement of solutes across a cell membrane against a concentration gradient (i.e., from an area of lower concentration to an area of higher concentration); energy—in the form of adenosine triphosphate (ATP)—expended by cell
   1. Sodium-potassium pump: major active transport system in cell membrane, sodium moved from ICF into ECF, potassium moved from ECF into ICF
   2. Other examples of solutes delivered to the cell by active transport: calcium, hydrogen, and glucose

See text pages
_____

III. Fluid balance: In health, intake equals output; anions equal cations.

A. Fluid intake: sources of water, average adult intake 2600 ml/day
   1. Fluids: largest source of water; intake varies with environmental temperature, activity level, diet (e.g., amount of salt in food); average adult intake 1300 ml/day
   2. Food: much has high water content (e.g., fruit); average adult intake 1000 ml/day
   3. Metabolism: water is a by-product of metabolic activity of cell (oxidation); average adult production 300 ml/day

B. Fluid output: avenues of water loss, average adult output 2600 ml/day
   1. Kidneys: largest avenue of water loss; urine output varies with amount of fluid ingested, amount of solutes excreted, and losses from other sources (e.g., perspiration); adult average output 1500 ml/day
   2. Skin: water lost 2 ways
      a) Insensible perspiration: loss of water through diffusion, independent of intake, client unaware of loss, average adult output 450 ml/day
      b) Sensible perspiration: loss of water by sweating; amount varies with environmental temperature and activity; client aware of loss; average adult output 150 ml/day, but can increase to 3.5 liters/day with heavy activity
   3. Lungs: loss of water as expired vapor, insensible loss, independent of intake, average adult output 300 ml/day
   4. Gastrointestinal tract: loss of water through feces, average adult output 200 ml/day
      a) Most fluid in gastrointestinal tract is resorbed.
      b) Abnormal conditions (e.g., diarrhea, fistula) cause serious loss of fluids and electrolytes from gastrointestinal system.

C. Regulation of intake and output: essential to health; rapid, sensitive control mechanisms
   1. Thirst: desire to drink, major regulator of intake (see Nurse Alert, "Factors Abnormally Affecting Thirst")
      a) Osmoreceptors: cells in the hypothalamus that are stimulated by an increase in osmotic pressure to initiate thirst (e.g., People feel thirsty after eating salty potato chips because increased electrolyte levels [NaCl] cause increase in osmotic pressure.)
      b) Decreased extracellular fluid volume
      c) Dry mouth: decreased salivary output; stimulates thirst; may be caused by conditions unrelated to dehydration (e.g., drugs like atropine)

Factors Abnormally Affecting Thirst

The thirst response may be triggered with abnormal frequency or the response itself may be altered:

- By age—In clients older than 60 years, osmoreceptors are less sensitive to increasing osmolality.
- By disease states—Polydipsia (frequent drinking due to extreme thirst) is symptomatic of conditions such as diabetes mellitus, diabetes insipidus, and hypoglycemia.
- By high fever—Resulting dehydration stimulates excessive thirst.
- By certain medications—Dry mouth, a common side effect of many medications, may stimulate polydipsia.
- By altered states of consciousness—Certain narcotic drugs may depress the response of osmoreceptors.
- By mental state—Mental or cognitive impairment may stimulate polydipsia or produce insensitivity to thirst cues.

2. Hormones affecting kidney function: The kidney is the major regulator of volume and concentration of output.
   a) Antidiuretic hormone (ADH): produced by hypothalamus and stored by pituitary, released in response to increased osmotic pressure in extracellular fluid (see Nurse Alert, "Pathological Changes in Antidiuretic Hormone Production")
      (1) Increased ADH production results in increased water resorption from distal tubules of kidney.
      (2) Renal output (urine volume) is decreased.

Pathological Changes in Antidiuretic Hormone Production

Production of excess antidiuretic hormone—leading to decreased urine output and fluid imbalance—can have a wide variety of causes, including:

- Head trauma (injury or surgery)
- Certain drugs, including barbiturates, antineoplastic drugs, and nonsteroidal anti-inflammatory drugs
- Anesthesia and surgery (in general)
- Tumors of brain or lung, especially oat cell carcinoma of the lung

Production of antidiuretic hormone can be reduced or stopped—leading to greatly increased urine output and excessive thirst (diabetes insipidus) with high risk of fluid imbalance—as a result of:

- Head trauma (injury or surgery)
- Brain tumor
- Infection

        (3) Extracellular fluid volume is restored.

        (4) Osmotic pressure of extracellular fluid is decreased.

    b) Aldosterone: produced by adrenal cortex in response to low intravascular fluid volume, low plasma sodium, or high plasma potassium

        (1) Increased aldosterone production results in increased sodium (and water) resorption from distal tubules of kidney; large amounts of potassium are excreted.

        (2) Renal output is decreased.

        (3) Extracellular fluid volume is increased.

    c) Renin: produced by juxtaglomerular cells of kidney in response to decreased renal blood flow (low intravascular fluid volume)

        (1) Increased renin production results in peripheral vasoconstriction.

        (2) Renin production stimulates aldosterone production (see section III,C,2,b of this chapter for effects of aldosterone).

IV. Nursing process

See text pages
_____

A. Nursing assessment

  1. Obtain medical history relative to fluid and electrolyte balance.

    a) Disease process (e.g., diabetes mellitus, pancreatitis) or injury

    b) Medication (e.g., diuretics), including over-the-counter (OTC) or other therapy (e.g., total parenteral therapy [TPN])

    c) Abnormal fluid loss (e.g., large burn area, vomiting, diarrhea)

    d) Dietary restrictions (e.g., low sodium)

    e) Mobility restrictions as they affect access to fluids

    f) Recent fluid intake

    g) Use of alcohol or illegal drugs or both

  2. Obtain baseline vital signs, which provides basis to evaluate change.

    a) Temperature: Temperature elevation between 101°F and 103°F increases 24-hour fluid intake requirements by a minimum of 500 ml.

    b) Blood pressure: Comparison of supine and standing blood pressures provides a sensitive measure of fluid volume status.

    c) Central venous pressure: sensitive indicator of blood volume (as well as heart function and vascular tone); requires indwelling central venous catheter (in vena cava or right atrium); measured in cm of water, using a pressure manometer

    d) Pulse: Rapid, weak, or irregular pulse may indicate fluid and electrolyte imbalances.

    e) Weight: Infants and lean clients have a higher proportion of fluid to body weight than adults and obese clients have; rapid changes in weight reflect changes in body fluid volume (see Nurse Alert, "Weighing a Client to Monitor Fluid Volume Changes").

    f) Respiration: Excessive loss of fluid occurs with hyperventilation; irregular respiration may indicate electrolyte imbalance.

Clinical signs	Fluid and electrolyte imbalances
Temperature	
Elevated	Fluid volume deficit, sodium excess
Pulse	
Rapid	Sodium excess
Rapid, weak	Fluid volume deficit
Bounding, full	Extracellular fluid volume excess
Slow	Intracellular fluid volume excess
Respiration	
Rapid, deep	Metabolic acidosis
Moist rales	Extracellular fluid volume excess
Depressed	Metabolic alkalosis, magnesium excess
Blood pressure	
Hypotension	Sodium deficit, magnesium excess
Postural hypotension	Fluid volume deficit, potassium deficit
Hypertension	Fluid volume excess
Skin and mucous membranes	
Poor skin turgor	Fluid volume deficit
Dry, flushed skin	Sodium excess
Dry, swollen tongue	Sodium excess
Tight, smooth, shiny skin	Extracellular fluid volume excess
Warm, moist, flushed skin	Intracellular fluid volume excess
Skeletal muscles	
Muscle weakness	Potassium deficit, phosphorus deficit, sodium deficit
Flaccid paralysis	Potassium excess
Muscle cramps	Calcium deficit
Trousseau's sign	Calcium deficit
Chvostek's sign	Calcium deficit, magnesium deficit
Convulsions	Intracellular fluid volume excess, calcium deficit, magnesium deficit, phosphorus deficit

Figure 1–2
Selected Assessment Cues in Fluid and Electrolyte Imbalances

! NURSE *ALERT* !

Weighing a Client to Monitor Fluid Volume Changes

To ensure accurate determination of body weight when monitoring changes in total body fluid volume, the nurse should:

- Make certain that the scale is balanced; check the platform to make sure that it is not loose or wobbly.
- Use the same scale each time the client is weighed.
- Weigh the client in the morning before breakfast but after voiding.
- Make sure the client is wearing the same or similar-weight dry clothes for each weighing.

3. Assess intake and output: Establish baseline readings (see Client Teaching Checklist, "Points to Cover about Intake and Output").
   a) Measure intake fluids: liquids taken orally (including liquid foods), IV fluids, subcutaneous fluids, fluids used to irrigate drainage tubes, and enteral solutions and water given by feeding tube
      (1) Record time, amount, and type of all fluids.
      (2) Calibrate nonstandard vessels (e.g., hospital drinking glasses) to ensure accuracy.
   b) Measure output fluids: urine, vomitus, diarrhea, and drainage from fistulas, wounds, and/or gastric suction
      (1) Record time, amount, and type of all fluids.
      (2) Use small, calibrated measuring containers to accurately measure small outputs.
   c) Estimate other output fluids: unmeasured or spilled vomitus or diarrhea, incontinent urine, wound drainage, perspiration, prolonged hyperventilation (see Nurse Alert, "Common Mistakes in Measuring Intake and Output")
4. Assess physical signs.
   a) Edema: Pressing fingers into client's soft tissue leaves depression that gradually disappears.
   b) Skin turgor (elasticity): In normal client, pinched skin immediately falls back into place (not valid for elderly).
   c) Oral cavity: turgor of tongue, moisture in mouth, saliva output

✔ CLIENT TEACHING CHECKLIST ✔

Points to Cover about Intake and Output

Clients and their families often unintentionally alter intake-output measurements.

✔ Explain to the client and the client's family the reason for the intake-output measurements.
✔ Ask the client and the family to leave any urine or vomitus in its container until it can be measured.
✔ Ask the client to inform the nurse of any liquids (such as juice) that were intended for the client but were consumed by visitors.
✔ Ask the client and the family to indicate the volume of any fluids—for example, water or ice chips—served by the family (half the volume of ice chips should be counted as fluid).

    d) Appearance of skin

    e) Veins: neck vein filling (jugular venous pressure) measured noninvasively, hand vein filling estimated by observation

    f) Neuromuscular irritability: Chvostek's sign, Trousseau's sign, deep-tendon reflexes

    g) Speech and behavior

5. Assess laboratory test results: Normal ranges vary slightly from laboratory to laboratory; establish baseline.

    a) Tests on blood

       (1) Serum potassium: normal range 3.5–5.0 mEq/L; alterations in acid-base balance affect potassium levels; decreased values suggest metabolic alkalosis; increased values suggest acidosis

       (2) Serum sodium: normal range 135–145 mEq/L; closely related to body water status; increased values suggest body water deficit

       (3) Serum calcium: normal-range total calcium 4.5–5.5 mEq/L or 9–11 mg/dl, ionized calcium 2.2–2.5 mEq/L or 4.5–5.0 mg/dl; measurements influenced by pH are serum albumin, fatty acids, lactate, bicarbonate, citrate, and phosphate; some radiographic media

       (4) Serum magnesium: normal range 1.3–2.1 mEq/L; hemolysis of blood sample releases intracellular magnesium and invalidates results

       (5) Serum chloride: normal range 95–108 mEq/L; lower values suggest metabolic alkalosis; higher values may be associated with excess administration of isotonic saline

       (6) Serum carbon dioxide content: normal range 22–32 mEq/L; indicates degree of alkalinity or acidity of blood; lower values suggest metabolic acidosis

       (7) Serum phosphate: normal adult range 1.7–2.6 mEq/L; values higher in children; hemolysis of blood sample releases intracellular phosphate and invalidates results

      (8) Serum osmolality: normal range 280–295 mOsm/kg; higher values suggest body water deficit; lower values suggest body water excess

      (9) Anion gap: measures sodium minus the sum of chloride and bicarbonate ($Na^+ - [Cl^- + HCO_3^-]$); normal range 12 ±2 mEq/L; higher values suggest metabolic acidosis

    (10) Blood urea nitrogen (BUN): normal range 8–25 mg/dl; higher values suggest reduced renal flow secondary to fluid deficit; lower values suggest fluid excess

    (11) Creatinine: normal range 0.6–1.5 mg/dl; evaluates renal dysfunction

    (12) Hemoglobin: normal range male 13–18 g/dl, female 12–16 g/dl; lower values suggest fluid excess

    (13) Hematocrit: normal range male 44%–52%, female 39%–47%; indicates percentage of red blood cells in total blood volume; higher values suggest fluid deficit; lower values suggest fluid excess

    (14) Plasma lactate: normal range 0.3–1.3 mEq/L; values above 4–5 mEq/L suggest lactic acidosis

    (15) Albumin: normal range 3.5–4.8 g/dl; lower levels reduce colloid osmotic pressure, causing edema

  b) Tests on urine

      (1) Urinary sodium: normal range 40–220 mEq/24 hour; varies strongly with diet; evaluate in view of total clinical picture

      (2) Urinary potassium: normal range 25–125 mEq/24 hour; used to assess hormonal functioning and to determine whether hypokalemia is of renal or nonrenal origin

      (3) Urinary chloride: normal range 110–250 mEq/24 hour; varies with diet; usually similar to urinary sodium in hypovolemia (reduced blood volume), because sodium and chloride are resorbed together

      (4) Urinary calcium: normal adult range 50–300 g/24 hour; varies strongly with diet; higher values may suggest metastatic tumors

      (5) Specific gravity (SG): normal range 1.003–1.035; indicates state of hydration and solute load excreted; higher values suggest fluid deficit

      (6) Urinary pH: normal range 4.5–8.0; reflects serum pH; helps confirm presence of alkalosis or acidosis

 B. Nursing diagnoses

  1. Fluid volume deficit related to body fluid imbalance

  2. Fluid volume excess related to body fluid imbalance

  3. Altered urinary elimination related to body fluid imbalance

C. Nursing interventions: Look for changes and trends.
  1. Monitor vital signs, including daily weights: Report abnormal vital signs or changes from baseline (see section IV,A,2 of this chapter for information on vital signs).
  2. Monitor intake and output: Report output of less than 700 ml/24 hours or greater than 2000 ml/24 hours or significant changes in intake or output (see section IV,A,3 of this chapter for information on monitoring intake and output).
  3. Check osmolality of IV fluids: Continued use of hypo-osmolar or hyperosmolar IV fluids may cause fluid and electrolyte imbalances.
  4. Check laboratory test results for changes from baseline levels: Report significant changes (see section IV,A,5 of this chapter for information on laboratory tests).

1. If a client has an excess of fluid in the interstitial space, which of the following is the nurse most likely to find on assessment?
   a. Poor skin turgor
   b. Distended neck veins
   c. Peripheral edema
   d. Elevated blood pressure

2. During a heat wave, the age group that is at highest risk for fluid volume deficits is:
   a. Infants.
   b. School-age children.
   c. Adolescents.
   d. Middle-aged adults.

3. A client's leg got crushed yesterday in a farm accident. The nurse must monitor the client for a dangerous increase in serum levels of:
   a. Bicarbonate.
   b. Calcium.
   c. Potassium.
   d. Sodium.

4. A client sustained a head injury that reduced secretion of antidiuretic hormone (ADH) by the pituitary gland. It is critical that the nurse monitor the client for:
   a. Elevated serum potassium levels.
   b. Peripheral edema.
   c. High blood pressure.
   d. Excessive urine output.

5. Which of the following would be an appropriate etiology for a nursing diagnosis of fluid volume excess?
   a. Deficient cortisol secretion
   b. Suppression of parathyroid function
   c. Deficient renin production
   d. Excessive aldosterone secretion

6. Which of the following assessment findings is associated with fluid volume deficit?
   a. Urine specific gravity = 1.025
   b. Tachycardia
   c. Single longitudinal furrow in tongue
   d. Flushed, warm skin

7. Which of the following nursing actions is likely to improve the accuracy of intake records?
   a. Documenting the exact volume of ice chips consumed as fluid intake
   b. Asking family members to indicate on the intake record any fluids the client drinks
   c. Listing as intake the volumes of all empty fluid containers on the tray
   d. Estimating how much the client has taken when only part of the container is consumed

8. A 35-year-old client weighs 154 lb (70 kg). In an evaluation of the client's output during an 8-hour shift, which of the following urine volumes should the nurse consider to be abnormal?
   a. 150 ml
   b. 300 ml
   c. 850 ml
   d. 1000 ml

9. The nurse should identify *high risk for intravascular fluid volume deficit* as a nursing diagnosis for the client who has low serum levels of:
   a. Calcium.
   b. Magnesium.
   c. Potassium.
   d. Sodium.

10. A client has an indwelling urinary catheter. Urine output has been 800–1000 ml/shift for 3 days. At 7 A.M. the nurse discovers that the drainage bag, which was last emptied at 11 P.M., contains only 100 ml of urine. The best action the nurse could take initially would be to:
    a. Report the decreased urinary output to the physician immediately.
    b. Document the output and alert the oncoming nurse to closely monitor the client's output.
    c. Check the catheter for kinking or other obstructions.

d. Encourage the client to increase his or her intake of water and juices.

11. A client had a thyroidectomy 3 days ago. The nurse should suspect that the parathyroid glands have been damaged by the surgery if the client develops:

   a. Hypokalemia.
   b. Hypocalcemia.
   c. Hypernatremia.
   d. Hyperchloremia.

12. Which of the following laboratory values is consistent with a fluid volume deficit?

   a. Hematocrit = 46%
   b. Serum osmolality = 305 mOsm/kg
   c. Urine specific gravity = 1.010
   d. Blood urea nitrogen = 6

ANSWERS

1. **Correct answer is c.** Edema is caused by accumulation of excess fluid between the cells (i.e., in the interstitial space).
   a. Poor skin turgor reflects a decrease, not an increase, in interstitial fluid.
   b and d. Both distension of the neck veins and elevated blood pressure indicate increased intravascular pressure, which may occur when there is increased intravascular fluid. These symptoms are not related to interstitial fluid status.

2. **Correct answer is a.** Infants have proportionately more body fluid than any other age group (70%–80% of body weight). More than half of a newborn's body fluid is in the extracellular compartment, from which it is readily lost from the body. Infants are dependent on others to meet their fluid needs.
   b, c, and d. All of these age groups are at lower risk than infants and the elderly. Body composition of a school-age child is the same as an adult's (about 60% water). All of these age groups can obtain their own fluids. By adolescence, only 20% of body fluid is extracellular.

3. **Correct answer is c.** In a crush injury, damaged cells release intracellular components into the extracellular compartment. Potassium is the major intracellular cation, but is normally present in only small amounts in the extracellular fluid. Release of large amounts of potassium from damaged cells into plasma can result in dangerous increases in serum potassium.
   b. Calcium is not a major component of intracellular fluid. Cell damage would not raise serum calcium levels.
   a and d. Bicarbonate and sodium levels are normally higher in extracellular fluid than in intracellular fluid. Cell damage would not raise serum bicarbonate or sodium levels.

4. **Correct answer is d.** ADH stimulates the kidneys to retain water. If the client's pituitary is secreting insufficient ADH, the client will lose body fluids through excessive urine output and may suffer a severe fluid volume deficit.
   a. Insufficient aldosterone secretion could produce elevated serum potassium levels. ADH does not directly affect serum potassium levels.
   b and c. Peripheral edema and high blood pressure both are associated with fluid retention. Both might occur with increased, but not decreased, ADH secretion.

5. **Correct answer is d.** Aldosterone acts on the kidney tubules to promote sodium reabsorption. When sodium is retained, fluid is also retained, and fluid volume excess may result.
   a. Cortisol promotes sodium and water retention. Excessive—not deficient—levels of cortisol would contribute to fluid volume excess.
   b. Parathyroid hormone affects calcium balance, not fluid balance.
   c. Renin stimulates the adrenal glands to secrete aldosterone. Deficient renin secretion would reduce aldosterone, causing fluid volume deficit, not fluid volume excess.

6. Correct answer is b. Tachycardia is often the first vital sign change due to decreased vascular volume.

a. This is a normal urine specific gravity (range = 1.003–1.035).
c. This is a normal finding. In fluid volume deficit the tongue shrinks and additional furrows appear.
d. Severe fluid volume deficit causes peripheral vasoconstriction, which results in cool, pale skin.

7. Correct answer is b. If family members are unaware of the need to record intake, they may fail to report fluids they give the client.

a. Water expands when it is frozen. Fluid intake from ice chips should be recorded as half the volume of ice chips consumed.
c. The nurse should not assume based on empty containers that the client has consumed fluid. The client should be asked what fluids were consumed.
d. Each estimate decreases the accuracy of the record. The actual amount consumed can be determined by measuring what remains in the container and subtracting it from the total the container had in it originally.

8. Correct answer is a. The normal range for urine output is 0.5–2.0 ml/kg/hour. During an 8-hour shift, a client's output should be between 280 and 1120 ml. An alternative rule of thumb is that 30 ml/hour of urine output is required to maintain adequate renal function. Under that rule, the client needs to excrete at least 240 ml in 8 hours.

b, c, and **d.** All of these amounts fall within the normal range.

9. Correct answer is d. Sodium is the primary electrolyte in extracellular fluid. Sodium provides a large portion of the osmotic force that holds fluid in the intravascular compartment. When sodium is deficient, fluid is lost from the vascular space.

a, b, and **c.** Calcium, magnesium, and potassium all are present in small amounts in extracellular fluid. They do not make significant contributions to the osmotic pressure that retains fluid in the vascular space.

10. Correct answer is c. Further assessment to identify the cause of the unusual finding is the best initial action. Impaired drainage of the catheter may be the cause of the low amount of drainage.

a and **d.** It would be inappropriate to take any action before determining the cause of the unusual finding.
b. Immediate intervention might be needed if urine output were really this low. Delaying for further monitoring could be dangerous.

11. Correct answer is b. Parathyroid hormone (PTH) raises calcium levels. Damage to the parathyroid glands would reduce available PTH, lowering calcium levels.

a and **c.** PTH does not affect sodium or potassium levels. Aldosterone or cortisol from the adrenal glands would alter these electrolytes.
d. Hyperchloremia is most often caused by excessive administration of IV saline. It is not related to PTH levels.

12. Correct answer is b. Serum osmolality is normally 280–295 mOsm/kg. Elevated serum osmolality reflects hemoconcentration—the result of intravascular fluid volume deficit.

a. This is a normal finding. Hematocrit would be elevated by fluid volume deficit.
c. This is a normal finding. Urine specific gravity is likely to be elevated in fluid volume deficit.
d. Normal blood urea nitrogen (BUN) range is 8–25 mg/dl. Fluid volume deficit may elevate BUN. Reduced BUN suggests fluid volume excess.

2

Fluid Volume Imbalances

NURSING HIGHLIGHTS

1. Fluid imbalances often are secondary to inadequate regulatory mechanisms, disease, or trauma; they cannot be considered without considering the underlying cause of the imbalance.
2. Fluid volume deficit is much more common than fluid volume excess; dehydration occurs most frequently in infants and the elderly.
3. With extracellular fluid volume shifts (third-space shifts), clients do not lose weight although the amount of fluid physiologically available to the body is decreased; clients gain weight when IV fluids are introduced to restore blood volume.

GLOSSARY

ascites—accumulation of serous fluid in the peritoneal cavity
hypervolemia—increase in the circulating volume of blood or vascular fluid
hypovolemia—decrease in the circulating volume of blood or vascular fluid

I. Fluid volume deficit (FVD)	II. Fluid volume excess (FVE)	III. Extracellular fluid volume shifts (third-space shifts)

See text pages
_____

I. Fluid volume deficit (FVD): can exist alone or with electrolyte imbalances; cause is excess fluid loss, inadequate fluid intake, or combination of excess output and inadequate intake (most common); although dehydration, technically, refers to loss of water only, that term is commonly used for FVD

A. Types of deficits
   1. Iso-osmolar FVD (isotonic dehydration): Water and electrolytes—primarily sodium—are lost in equal proportions.
      a) Serum electrolytes remain unchanged at 280–295 mOsm/L; serum remains iso-osmolar.
      b) Fluid loss comes mainly from the extracellular compartment.
      c) Iso-osmolar FVD is the most common type of dehydration.
   2. Hyperosmolar FVD (hypertonic dehydration): Water is lost in excess of the amount of sodium lost.
      a) Solutes increase in proportion to body water; serum becomes hyperosmolar.
      b) Serum osmolality rises above 295 mOsm/kg.
      c) Water is drawn from the cells (intracellular space) into the interstitial (tissue) space in response to an increase in sodium levels in the serum; intracellular dehydration results.
   3. Hypo-osmolar FVD (hypotonic dehydration): Sodium is lost in excess of the amount of water lost.
      a) Solutes are decreased in proportion to body water; serum becomes hypo-osmolar.
      b) Serum osmolality falls below 280 mOsm/L.
      c) Extracellular water is drawn into the cells, resulting in a decrease in extracellular fluid volume—especially blood volume—and intracellular fluid excess, or water intoxication.

B. Pathophysiology and etiology: nearly always related to abnormal fluid loss; rate increases when intake is decreased in conjunction with fluid loss; can develop FVD solely from decreased intake over time
   1. Loss of gastrointestinal fluids: Any condition that interferes with absorption of fluids from gastrointestinal tract can cause serious FVD; generally gastric fluids are iso-osmolar, with extracellular fluid.
      a) Vomiting: Prolonged loss of iso-osmolar gastric fluid causes iso-osmolar FVD; severe vomiting may lead to excess water loss and hyperosmolar FVD.
      b) Diarrhea: iso-osmolar fluid loss in 70% of clients is caused by decreased bowel absorption; other causes of diarrhea may result

in electrolyte imbalances; normally only 200 ml/day of water lost through feces; common cause of FVD in infants and children

   c) Gastrointestinal suction: iso-osmolar FVD

   d) Gastric fistulas and abscesses: iso-osmolar FVD

   e) Excessive laxative use: iso-osmolar FVD; usually accompanies eating disorders (e.g., anorexia, bulimia)

2. Polyuria: excessive excretion of urine; hyperosmolar FVD

   a) Condition occurs in clients with diabetes insipidus or diabetes mellitus (see Chapter 12 for information on diabetic ketoacidosis and nonketotic hyperosmolar coma) and in clients receiving hyperosmolar tube feedings.

   b) Serum becomes hyperosmolar when glucose, ketone bodies, protein, and/or electrolyte concentrations increase.

   c) Kidneys excrete large volume of urine in which water loss exceeds electrolyte loss.

3. Fever: iso-osmolar FVD

   a) Fever increases metabolism, resulting in increased metabolic wastes; additional fluid is required to remove wastes.

   b) Respiration is increased, resulting in increased water vapor loss through lungs.

4. Sweating: Sweat is hypo-osmolar, resulting in hyperosmolar FVD.

   a) Caused by fever or high environmental temperatures

   b) Profuse sweating accompanied by either sodium excess if no fluids are consumed or sodium deficit if excessive amounts of water are consumed (see Chapter 3, section II, for discussion of sodium imbalance)

5. Inadequate intake of fluids: hyperosmolar FVD

   a) Caused by nausea, anorexia, neurological impairment of swallowing mechanism, impaired swallowing due to oral or pharyngeal pain, limited access to fluids, or severe depression (see Nurse Alert, "Inadequate Intake in the Mobility Impaired")

   b) Abnormal functioning of thirst mechanism (see Chapter 1, section III,C,1, for a discussion of thirst)

6. Increased solute intake (e.g., salt, sugar, protein): hyperosmolar FVD; hyperosmolar serum constitutes a relative water deficit; water drawn

---

❗ NURSE _ALERT_ ❗

Inadequate Intake in the Mobility Impaired

In the absence of complicating factors, otherwise healthy clients whose mobility is impaired or who have pain or difficulty swallowing may develop long-term FVD resulting in permanent damage to the renal tubules. Such clients should have fluids presented to them in a modified fashion and be offered frequent assistance in drinking in order to compensate for their physical limitations. For clients with dysphagia, thickened liquids and slushes are safer and easier to swallow.

from cells causes intracellular dehydration; water is lost at a higher rate than solutes

C. Signs and symptoms
   1. Changes in weight: Rapid weight loss reflects loss of body fluids (1 liter of fluid weighs about 2 lb).
   2. Changes in skin
      a) Turgor: decreased
         (1) After being pinched, skin remains slightly elevated due to interstitial fluid deficit (not a reliable sign in the elderly, as skin turgor is lost with elasticity).
         (2) Decreased turgor is less pronounced in hyperosmolar FVD as fluid moves into interstitial spaces.
      b) Color: gray
      c) Temperature: cold in iso-osmolar and hypo-osmolar FVDs; cold or hot in hyperosmolar FVD
      d) Feel: dry in iso-osmolar FVD; clammy in hypo-osmolar FVD; thickened in hyperosmolar FVD
      e) Veins: Neck-vein filling drops, and hand-vein filling slows.
   3. Changes in oral cavity
      a) Tongue: turgor decreased; smaller, with longitudinal furrows due to loss of interstitial fluid (tongue furrowing not altered by age; reliable sign in the elderly)
      b) Mucous membranes: dry to parched in iso-osmolar and hyperosmolar FVDs; slightly moist in hypo-osmolar FVD; may also be dry because of mouth breathing
   4. Changes in vital signs
      a) Temperature: subnormal in iso-osmolar FVD (in absence of infection) due to decreased metabolism; elevated in hyperosmolar FVD
      b) Postural hypotension: Drop of 15 mm Hg or more when position changes from lying down to standing suggests inadequate intravascular volume.
      c) Blood pressure and pulse: Increase in pulse of 15 or more beats/minute suggests inadequate intravascular volume; as FVD becomes severe, blood pressure drops and heart rate increases to try to compensate for decreased intravascular fluid volume.
      d) Central venous pressure: less than 4 cm of water in vena cava, less than 0 cm of water in right atrium
      e) Respiration: Rate increases.
   5. Changes in urinary output: oliguria (inadequate urinary output)
      a) Inadequate perfusion of the kidneys results in reduced urine volume: Volume deficit of intravascular fluid brings inadequate plasma to glomeruli of kidneys.

b) Urine volume of less than 30 ml/hour in adult is cause for concern.

c) Persistent oliguria can cause renal tubule damage.

6. Changes in laboratory test results

    a) Urinary specific gravity: increases

    b) Hematocrit: increases

    c) Blood urea nitrogen (BUN)/creatinine ratio: BUN increases out of proportion to serum creatinine because of decreased glomerular filtration rate in long-standing FVDs.

7. Changes in behavior: irritable to lethargic in iso-osmolar FVD; lethargic to comatose and convulsions in hypo-osmolar FVD; lethargic with extreme hyperirritability in hyperosmolar FVD

D. Treatment and management: prompt treatment necessary to prevent renal damage

1. Oral replacement of fluids

    a) Oral route is preferred in mild to moderate FVD when client is alert and able to drink; offer fluids in glass or cup to sitting clients; turn supine client on side if possible.

    b) Water or other liquid that is attractive to client is best source of replacement fluids; offer small amounts frequently; infants, the elderly, and clients whose mobility is impaired may require assistance to drink.

    c) Antinausea medication may facilitate successful oral replacement of fluids.

2. Parenteral replacement of fluids: prescribed by physician, administered by nurse

    a) Fluids approximately iso-osmolar to extracellular fluid; water never given intravenously

    b) Examples of preferred replacement solutions

        (1) Lactated Ringer's: electrolyte content similar to normal blood serum; replenishes extracellular fluid volume

        (2) Normal saline solution (0.9% sodium chloride [NaCl]): replaces fluid and sodium loss

        (3) 5% hydrated dextrose (D_5W) in water: replaces water deficit; aids in increasing urine output; dextrose is metabolized rapidly leaving a hypo-osmolar solution (see Chapter 5, section II,A,1, for cautions on the use of D_5W)

    c) Rate of administration of intravenous fluids influences value of fluids to client; fluids given over a period of 12–24 hours safest and most effective; rate prescribed by physician, administered by nurse

E. Nursing process

1. Nursing assessment: frequently involves evaluating changes in assessment factors through time

    a) Assess client history for factors related to FVD (e.g., vomiting, diarrhea, disease, medication).

    b) Assess skin for turgor, dryness, color, and condition of mucous membranes.

c) Check vital signs, specifically, temperature, blood pressure (first sitting, then standing), weight, pulse, and respiration.

d) Check urine for output and concentration.

2. Nursing diagnoses: Many cases of FVD require collaborative or interdependent evaluation; the nurse monitors the client and collaborates with the physician rather than reaching an independent nursing diagnosis.

a) FVD related to inadequate intake, vomiting, diarrhea, or hemorrhage

b) Altered renal perfusion related to decreased blood flow and poor urinary output secondary to FVD

c) Altered oral mucous membranes related to FVD

d) High risk for impaired skin integrity related to FVD in body tissues

3. Nursing interventions

a) Monitor vital signs and compare with baseline: Frequency depends on severity of FVD.

b) Monitor intake and output: Frequency depends on severity of FVD.

c) Start oral replacement therapy: Frequently offer appropriate liquids in small quantities; assist client with drinking, as necessary.

d) Initiate parenteral replacement therapy if ordered: Monitor rate of administration of replacement fluid; maintain sterility of solution.

e) Report inadequate response: Prompt replacement therapy is necessary to prevent renal damage.

f) Monitor elderly clients and clients with renal or cardiac problems for volume overload during aggressive fluid replacement therapy.

g) Monitor condition of skin and mucous membranes.

h) Offer frequent oral care.

i) Turn and massage client frequently to prevent skin breakdown.

j) Monitor body weight: Loss of 1 kg equals loss of 1000 ml fluid.

k) Monitor changes in laboratory test results.

See text pages
_____

II. Fluid volume excess (FVE): retention of excess fluid in the body; often occurs in conjunction with renal failure; electrolytes may also be out of balance

A. Types of excesses

1. Extracellular FVE: edema (peripheral or pulmonary); abnormal retention of fluids in the interstitial space; secondary to increase in body sodium

a) Percent adult body weight that is water can increase from 60% (normal) to 69%–72% (edema).

b) Interstitial fluid increases from about 15% (normal) to about 28% of body weight.

c) Water and sodium are retained in approximately the same proportions as in normal extracellular fluid.

d) Serum sodium concentration remains near normal.

2. Intracellular FVE: water intoxication; abnormal retention of fluid within cells; results from an excess of water and/or decrease in solutes in vascular system

a) Serum osmolality of vascular fluid is decreased.

b) Hypo-osmolar fluid in vascular system moves by osmosis into cells (from area of lesser solute concentration to area of greater solute concentration).

c) Affected cells swell (cellular edema); cerebral cells are usually the first to be affected.

B. Pathophysiology and etiology: usually related to compromised regulatory mechanisms; compounded by overzealous administration of fluids and ingestion of excess sodium in diet

1. Physiological factors leading to extracellular FVE: One or more of these factors underlie clinical manifestations of edema.

a) Increased plasma hydrostatic pressure in capillaries: Blood dammed in venous system raises capillary pressure (e.g., in congestive heart failure); increased pressure forces fluid into interstitial space.

b) Decreased plasma colloidal osmotic pressure: caused by decreased plasma protein levels (e.g., in malnutrition); water flows out of capillaries and into interstitial space

c) Increased capillary permeability: Plasma proteins leak out of capillaries into interstitial space more rapidly than they can be returned by lymphatic system (e.g., in bacterial infection).

d) Increased sodium retention: caused by failure of kidney to regulate level of sodium ions in extracellular fluid (e.g., inadequate blood flow, diseased kidneys)

e) Decreased lymphatic drainage: reduces return of proteins to circulatory system (e.g., cancer of lymph system, surgical removal of lymph nodes); leads to decrease in plasma colloidal osmotic pressure

2. Common etiology of edema

a) Failure of regulatory mechanisms: congestive heart failure, renal failure, or steroid excess (Cushing's syndrome)

b) Disease: cirrhosis of the liver, cancer of lymph system, or bacterial infection

c) Trauma: burns, fractures, or surgery

d) Human factors: excess administration of sodium-containing fluids (e.g., 0.9% NaCl or lactated Ringer's) or excess ingestion of sodium in diet (see Client Teaching Checklist, "Dietary Sources of Sodium")

3. Major conditions causing intracellular FVE (water intoxication): less common than extracellular FVE
   a) Either excessive intake of plain water with few solutes or excessive use of hypo-osmolar IV solutions (e.g., 0.45% NaCl, D_5W [D_5W is iso-osmolar, but dextrose is rapidly metabolized, leaving plain water]) dilutes vascular fluid.
   b) Deficit of electrolytes and proteins creates hypo-osmolar vascular fluid: malnutrition, diet low in electrolytes, or irrigation of nasogastric tube with plain water
   c) Syndrome of inappropriate antidiuretic hormone (SIADH) causes massive resorption of water by kidneys: stress, surgery, trauma, certain drugs, anesthesia, or brain or lung tumors
   d) Kidney dysfunction decreases water excretion: renal impairment

C. Signs and symptoms
   1. Peripheral edema: extracellular FVE with swelling in the extremities
      a) Pitting edema in extremities: Finger indentation remains when finger pressed into edematous tissue; presence in morning may indicate inadequate heart, liver, or kidney function.
      b) Changes in vital signs: rapid weight increase; central venous pressure greater than 11 cm of water in vena cava and greater than 4 cm of water in right atrium; bounding, full pulse
      c) Skin: tight and shiny over edematous area
      d) Face: puffy eyelids

✔ CLIENT TEACHING CHECKLIST ✔

Dietary Sources of Sodium

Clients who are on sodium-restricted diets should be made aware of the following sources of dietary sodium.

✔ Sodium added as a preservative in processed foods such as bacon, pickled foods, and luncheon meats
✔ Sodium added as seasoning in canned foods such as canned soup
✔ So-called hidden sodium from baking powder in baked goods
✔ Sodium exchanged for other ions in household water softeners
✔ Sodium in over-the-counter drugs such as Alka-Seltzer
✔ Sodium occurring naturally in the drinking water of some communities

e) Laboratory test results: decreased BUN, hematocrit, serum protein, and albumin (due to plasma dilution); decreased serum osmolality (less than 275 mOsm/kg)

2. Pulmonary edema: extracellular FVE, in which alveoli of lungs fill with fluid
   a) Constant, irritated cough: often first clinical symptom
   b) Dyspnea (difficulty breathing) and orthopnea (breathing easier when sitting or standing): due to fluid in lungs
   c) Decreased tolerance for activity
   d) Moist rales in lungs: due to fluid congestion; heard with stethoscope
   e) Veins: neck veins engorged; peripheral veins of the hand slow to empty

3. Water intoxication: intracellular FVE
   a) Early signs: headache, nausea, vomiting, rapid weight gain, excessive sweating, and fingerprint edema over flat bony areas such as sternum and sacrum; cerebral cells affected first
   b) Neurologic signs: behavioral changes, irritability, disorientation, confusion, progressive apprehension, incoordination, drowsiness, and blurred vision; caused by swollen cerebral cells
   c) Changes in vital signs: increased blood pressure, intracranial pressure, and respiration rate; decreased pulse; vital sign changes are the reverse of those seen in clients with shock
   d) Late signs: warm, moist, flushed skin; muscle twitching; projectile vomiting; delirium; and convulsions, followed by coma

D. Treatment and management: Reduce excess water in body; primary therapy is to treat underlying cause (e.g., compromised regulatory mechanism, malnutrition, infection).
   1. Reduce water intake: Reducing water intake will not normally reduce extracellular FVE (edema), but it is effective in mild cases of intracellular FVE (water intoxication); water may be restricted in cases of renal failure.
   2. Reduce sodium intake: Low-sodium diet reduces water retention.
   3. Increase urine output: Diuretics promote urine flow by inhibiting salt and water resorption from kidney tubules; they often have undesirable effect on electrolyte balance.
   4. Increase osmolality of extracellular fluid (with intracellular FVE only): Lactated Ringer's or normal saline may be given; concentrated saline may be used for severe water intoxication, but may lead to edema.

E. Nursing process
   1. Nursing assessment: Assess for presence or worsening of FVE.
      a) Assess client history for underlying factors related to FVE (e.g., renal or cardiac insufficiency).
      b) Check vital signs: blood pressure, pulse, and weight; obtain baseline data
      c) Assess respiration and breath sounds.
      d) Assess peripheral-hand-vein emptying.

  e) Assess skin and tissue for peripheral pitting edema.

  f) Check urine output.

  g) Make dietary assessment relative to sodium intake.

  h) Assess for behavioral and neurological changes.

2. Nursing diagnoses: Many cases of FVE require collaborative or interdependent evaluation; the nurse monitors the client and collaborates with the physician rather than reaching an independent nursing diagnosis.

  a) FVE: edema related to body fluid overload secondary to heart, renal, or liver dysfunction

  b) Ineffective breathing patterns related to increased capillary permeability (pulmonary edema)

  c) Altered skin integrity related to edematous tissue (peripheral edema)

  d) FVE: water intoxication related to excessive infusion of hypo-osmolar solutions

  e) High risk for injury related to cerebral edema secondary to intracellular FVE

3. Nursing interventions

  a) Monitor vital signs and compare with baseline signs.

  b) Monitor fluid intake and output.

  c) Monitor weight daily for rapid changes.

  d) Monitor breathing patterns for changes in chest sounds and respiration.

  e) Administer diuretics, if ordered; monitor client response.

  f) Monitor laboratory test results for changes pertinent to electrolyte balance and fluid status.

  g) Monitor diet; instruct client in food selection.

  h) Monitor for worsening of underlying cause of FVE.

  i) Monitor parenteral fluid replacement if given (intracellular FVE).

  j) Monitor for changes in behavior indicating changes in neurological status (intracellular FVE).

See text pages

III. Extracellular fluid volume shifts (third-space shifts): Extracellular fluids become isolated in interstitial spaces in the body where they are unavailable for vascular functions.

A. Description

1. Large amounts of intravascular fluid shift from the vascular system into interstitial space; shift occurs, at least in part, through increased capillary permeability.

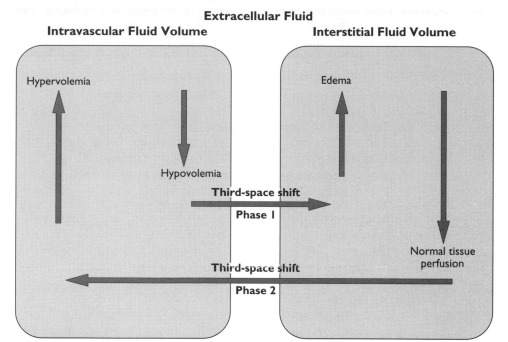

Extracellular Fluid

Intravascular Fluid Volume   Interstitial Fluid Volume

Hypervolemia   Edema

Hypovolemia

Third-space shift

Phase I

Normal tissue
perfusion

Third-space shift

Phase 2

Figure 2–1
Extracellular Fluid Movement during Third-Space Shift

    a) Location of third space may be either localized to single organ or area (e.g., abdomen, area around joint) or generalized throughout body (generalized edema).

    b) Fluid is physiologically nonfunctional and cannot be exchanged with other extracellular fluid in the body.

    c) Fluid losses cannot be observed or measured.

2. As a result of fluid shift to interstitial space, blood volume drops; functional FVD develops.

    a) Differs from FVD due to other causes because fluid remains in the body, although it is functionally lost.

    b) There is no corresponding loss of weight or observable excessive loss of fluid, as with vomiting or diarrhea.

3. Two phases characterize third-space shifts.

    a) Phase 1: movement of fluid out of vascular system and into interstitial space

        (1) Body attempts to compensate for decreased blood volume; renal tubules increase sodium and water resorption.

        (2) Symptoms of FVD develop.

        (3) Phase 1 may persist for a period ranging from 48 hours to several days, depending on cause.

      b) Phase 2: resorption of fluid from interstitial space back into vascular system
        (1) Symptoms of FVE can develop.
        (2) Duration of phase 2 is always longer than that of phase 1—often days.
        (3) Resorption may occur so slowly that no signs of FVE develop.

B. Pathophysiology and etiology
  1. Underlying physiological mechanism of extracellular fluid volume shift generally involves increased capillary permeability due to injury, inflammation, or ischemia; intravascular fluid leaks into interstitial space.
  2. By means of sodium and water conservation, body attempts to compensate for loss of fluid to third space.
  3. Common situations induce third-space shifts.
    a) Trauma and surgery: Fluid collects at site of trauma (e.g., blister, surgical incision); large amounts of fluids may be involved (up to 2–3 liters during extensive abdominal surgery; shift occurs immediately, reaching maximum in 5–6 hours.
    b) Burns: Third space takes the form of generalized edema; greatest shift occurs during first 8 hours.
    c) Intestinal obstruction: 6 liters or more of fluid may shift to interstitial space in lumen and wall of gut; functional FVD may be severe.
    d) Inflammatory lesions of organs in the abdominal cavity: Fluid shifts into peritoneum, bowel wall, and other tissues.
    e) Sepsis: produces generalized capillary leakage throughout body
    f) Pancreatitis: Loss of 30%–40% of plasma volume within 6 hours is possible.
    g) Ascites: associated with hepatic cirrhosis; fluid may accumulate slowly in peritoneal cavity without causing functional FVD, but third-space-shift problems occur if fluid rapidly reaccumulates following mechanical removal by paracentesis

C. Signs and symptoms
  1. Phase 1: Symptoms are similar to FVD and mimic shock symptoms.
    a) Vital signs: tachycardia and hypotension; effective blood volume is reduced
    b) Urine volume: less than 30 ml/hour; decreased plasma volume causes reduced renal perfusion
    c) Skin: poor skin and tongue turgor
    d) Central venous pressure: low; postural hypotension
    e) Laboratory test results: hematocrit elevated; high urinary specific gravity; urinary osmolality increased
    f) No weight loss as in FVD from other causes

2. Phase 2: Symptoms are those of FVE; often resorption of fluid is gradual, and minimal signs of FVE are observed.
   a) Vital signs: bounding pulse, elevated systolic blood pressure
   b) Urine volume: polyuria (as much as 200 ml/hour)
   c) Lungs: moist lung sounds, shortness of breath
   d) Central venous pressure: elevated; neck veins distended
   e) Laboratory test results: urinary specific gravity and osmolality decreased
   f) Measurable weight loss: fluid now physically removed from the body

D. Treatment and management
   1. Phase 1: Goal is to prevent damage to renal tubules due to fluid volume deficiency.
      a) Treat for fluid volume deficiency by increasing available fluids.
      b) IV fluids may be necessary to increase plasma volume.
   2. Phase 2: Goal is to avoid fluid overload as third-space fluids are reabsorbed into vascular system.
      a) Reduce fluid intake.
      b) Diuretics may aid in clearing excess intravascular fluid.

E. Nursing process
   1. Phase 1: Assess, monitor, and intervene as for FVD (same as section I,E of this chapter).
   2. Phase 2: Assess, monitor, and intervene as for FVE (same as section II,E of this chapter).

1. Which of the following clients should the nurse identify as being at highest risk for a hyperosmolar fluid volume deficit?

   a. A 6-year-old with gastroenteritis who has diarrhea
   b. A 45-year-old who has been vomiting for 8 hours
   c. A 25-year-old who is working outdoors in 95° weather
   d. A 92-year-old with a fever

2. Which of the following is most likely to be a reliable sign of a fluid volume deficit in an elderly client?

   a. Poor skin turgor
   b. Shrunken, furrowed tongue
   c. Elevated blood urea nitrogen
   d. Subnormal temperature

3. A client who has diabetes mellitus has had poor oral intake and an elevated blood glucose for 3 days. As a result of polyuria and reduced intake of fluids, the client now has a fluid volume deficit. Appropriate nursing diagnoses for this client include:

   a. High risk for impaired skin integrity related to decreased fluid in body tissues.
   b. High risk for ineffective breathing pattern related to increased exhalation of water vapor.
   c. Suprapubic pain related to irritation of bladder by highly concentrated urine.
   d. Altered thought processes related to shifting of fluid into brain cells.

4. Which of the following nursing outcomes would indicate that treatment for a fluid volume deficit has been effective?

   a. Urine output is 200 ml during an 8-hour shift.
   b. Client gains 1 lb in 24 hours.
   c. Urine specific gravity increases.
   d. Absence of pedal edema.

5. Which of the following would be an appropriate etiology for a nursing diagnosis of fluid volume excess: water intoxication?

   a. Increased production of antidiuretic hormone (ADH) stimulated by surgery and anesthetic drugs
   b. Frequent irrigations of the nasogastric tube with normal saline solution
   c. Increased hydrostatic pressure secondary to congestive heart failure
   d. Low serum protein levels secondary to impaired liver function

6. Which of the following assessment findings suggests a fluid volume excess?

   a. Bounding radial pulse
   b. Tenting when skin turgor is tested
   c. Serum sodium level higher than 145 mEq/L
   d. Central venous pressure (CVP) in the vena cava greater than 4 cm of water

7. Which of the following nursing diagnoses is most likely to be identified for a client with an extracellular fluid volume excess?

   a. Acute confusion related to shifting of fluid into cerebral cells
   b. High risk for injury related to sudden drop of blood pressure with position change
   c. Pain in legs related to intermittent muscle cramping
   d. Ineffective breathing pattern related to excess interstitial fluid in lungs

8. A low-sodium diet is prescribed to help reduce a client's fluid volume excess. Which of the following would be the best snack for this client?

   a. Half a bologna sandwich
   b. Bowl of canned mushroom soup
   c. Cup of corn flakes with skim milk
   d. Fresh apple slices

9. A client is admitted to the emergency room with a suspected intestinal obstruction. Because treatment has not yet been initiated, for which fluid imbalance is it most important that the nurse assess the client?

   a. Intracellular dehydration
   b. Third spacing of fluid
   c. Intravascular fluid volume excess
   d. Water intoxication

10. To detect complications of the second phase of a third-space fluid shift, the nurse should monitor the client for:

    a. High urine specific gravity.
    b. Postural hypotension.
    c. Elevated systolic blood pressure.
    d. Elevated hematocrit.

11. A client suffered a fractured hip this morning and is awaiting surgical repair. Which assessment tool would be most useful in monitoring the client for third spacing of fluids?

    a. Checking for weight changes
    b. Observing for temperature alterations
    c. Recording urinary output
    d. Auscultating breath sounds

12. A client is admitted to the hospital for treatment of a large pleural effusion. The client is hypotensive and oliguric. With which of the following IV fluids should the nurse anticipate treatment?

    a. A solution of 5% dextrose in water
    b. A balanced electrolyte solution
    c. Half-strength saline
    d. A colloid solution

ANSWERS

---

1. **Correct answer is c.** This client will sweat profusely, losing hypo-osmolar fluid.

   a. Most cases of diarrhea produce iso-osmolar fluid volume deficits.

   b. Gastric fluid lost in vomiting is iso-osmolar. Prolonged vomiting might cause excess water loss.
   d. Fever produces iso-osmolar fluid volume deficits.

2. **Correct answer is b.** Tongue furrowing remains a reliable sign of reduced tissue turgor in the elderly. It is not likely to be caused by other conditions.

   a. Decreased subcutaneous fat causes poor skin turgor even in well-hydrated elderly persons.
   c. The elderly commonly have some reduction of kidney function, which may elevate blood urea nitrogen, even without fluid volume deficit.
   d. Slower metabolism results in subnormal temperatures in the elderly, making such temperatures a less reliable sign of fluid volume deficit.

3. **Correct answer is a.** Polyuria and poor intake both produce hyperosmolar fluid volume deficit, causing fluid to shift out of body cells. This increases the risk of tissue breakdown.

   b. Excessive loss of water vapor does not alter breathing pattern.
   c. Urine becomes more concentrated as the kidneys try to conserve fluid. This is not usually painful.
   d. Fluid shifts into brain cells when a hypo-osmolar fluid volume deficit is present. In this client's case, fluid would shift out of tissue cells.

4. **Correct answer is b.** Weight gain of 1 lb in 24 hours correlates with a gain of approximately 500 ml of body fluid.

   a. This would reflect an output of 25 ml/hour and inadequate treatment.
   c. Increasing urine specific gravity would reflect worsening fluid volume deficit.
   d. Because pedal edema is not a sign of fluid volume deficit, its absence does not reflect effective treatment.

5. **Correct answer is a.** The stress of surgery and the effects of anesthetics increase ADH production, promoting retention of water. The resulting hypo-osmolar fluid volume excess shifts fluid into cells, causing water intoxication.

   b. Frequent irrigations with water could cause hypo-osmolar fluid volume excess. Saline is appropriate for irrigations.
   c. An intravascular fluid volume excess would increase hydrostatic pressure, causing edema.
   d. Decreased serum protein reduces osmotic pressure in the intravascular space. This results in a net movement of water into the interstitial space, causing edema.

6. **Correct answer is a.** A full, bounding pulse suggests increased intravascular volume and commonly occurs with extracellular fluid volume excess.

   b. This reflects poor skin turgor—a sign of fluid volume deficit.
   c. High sodium intake can contribute to fluid volume excess. However, the retained fluid dilutes the extra sodium, so serum sodium levels either remain the same or decrease. High serum sodium levels suggest body water deficit.
   d. CVP in the vena cava should be between 4 and 11 cm of water (0–4 cm of water in the right atrium). Fluid volume excess raises the CVP in the vena cava above 11 cm of water (above 4 cm of water in the right atrium).

7. **Correct answer is d.** Pulmonary edema occurs when intravascular pressure is elevated. Pulmonary edema produces dyspnea and orthopnea.

   a. This would be an appropriate nursing diagnosis in water intoxication.
   b. This nursing diagnosis reflects postural hypotension, which occurs in fluid volume deficit.
   c. Muscle cramping is associated with hypocalcemia.

8. **Correct answer is d.** Most fresh fruits and vegetables are low in sodium, making them good snacks for a client on a sodium-restricted diet.

   a, b, and **c.** Processed foods (like bologna), canned foods, dry cereals, and milk are relatively high in sodium. They would not be good choices for a client on a low-sodium diet.

9. **Correct answer is b.** In an acute intestinal obstruction, 6 liters or more of fluid can shift into the gut.

   a. Intravascular fluid volume deficit is the greatest concern during the first phase of third spacing.
   c. Once treatment has corrected the obstruction and fluid begins to shift back to the vascular space, an intravascular fluid volume excess may occur.
   d. Water intoxication is not likely, because the fluid shifting to the gut is most likely iso-osmolar, leaving the vascular space iso-osmolar.

10. **Correct answer is c.** High systolic blood pressure indicates hypervolemia, which may occur in the second phase of third spacing, when fluid shifts back into circulation.

    a. High specific gravity reflects concentration of urine, which occurs as the kidneys compensate for low vascular volume in the first phase of a fluid shift.
    b. Postural hypotension is indicative of the low vascular volume that characterizes the first phase of third spacing.
    d. Elevated hematocrit occurs with hemoconcentration in the first phase of a third-space fluid shift.

11. **Correct answer is c.** During the first 24 hours, fluid shifts from the intravascular space to the injured site, producing signs and symptoms of fluid volume deficit. Urinary output will be reduced, often falling below 30 ml/hour.

a. The weight does not change, because the fluid remains in the body when a third-space fluid shift occurs.

b. Temperature changes do not occur early in fluid volume deficit. An inflammatory response may elevate the client's temperature, masking this sign.

d. During the second phase of third spacing, this client could develop fluid volume excess with pulmonary edema. The client is in the first phase at this time.

12. **Correct answer is b.** Because the fluid shifted to the pleural space is iso-osmolar, an isotonic balanced electrolyte solution would be used to replace it.

a and **c.** Hypotonic solutions could cause significant hyponatremia if used to treat an iso-osmolar fluid shift.

d. Colloid solutions are used when the pathology includes protein depletion (e.g., burns, peritonitis). This is not the case with pleural effusion.

3

Specific Electrolyte Imbalances

NURSING HIGHLIGHTS

1. Electrolyte concentrations are regulated mainly by diet, absorption from the gastrointestinal tract, and resorption/excretion by the renal tubules in response to hormonal and chemical changes in the body.
2. Changes in electrolyte concentrations result in changes in the distribution of water in various fluid compartments of the body.
3. Many electrolyte imbalances are symptoms of underlying diseases such as cancers, renal disease, or hormonal imbalances.

4. Several electrolyte imbalances may occur simultaneously, thereby complicating treatment.
5. When correcting an electrolyte imbalance by the administration of parenteral fluids, one must use extreme care to prevent undesirable—possibly fatal—side effects, as the body is very sensitive to rapid changes in electrolyte levels.

GLOSSARY

anorexia nervosa—neurotic loss of appetite and unwillingness to eat, accompanied by weight loss

bulimia—condition characterized by recurring bouts of eating voraciously, usually followed by some form of purging such as self-induced vomiting, laxative abuse, or diuretic abuse

diabetes insipidus—excretion of large volumes of dilute urine as the result of insufficient antidiuretic hormone production or failure of the kidney to respond to the hormone

fingerprint edema—sufficient water retention in tissue to allow a finger pressed into the tissue to leave its mark when removed

paresthesia—spontaneous, abnormal sensation such as tingling or numbness, often on the face or in the extremities

tetany—intermittent muscular contractions accompanied by tremors, nerve tingling, and muscular pain; hands are usually first affected followed by face and trunk

ENHANCED OUTLINE

I. Electrolytes: substances that dissolve in water into electrically charged parts; major regulators of all body functions

See text pages

A. Cations and anions: See Chapter 1, section I,C,1, for a review of anions and cations.

B. Physiologic role of electrolytes: Most electrolytes have more than one function; often several electrolytes work together to mediate chemical events.
   1. Maintain electroneutrality in fluid compartments
   2. Mediate enzyme reactions (e.g., adenosine triphosphate [ATP] production)
   3. Alter cell membrane permeability
   4. Regulate nerve impulse transmission
   5. Regulate muscle contraction and relaxation
   6. Influence blood-clotting time

See text pages

II. Sodium (Na) imbalances: common in clinical practice; estimated minimum adult requirement 500 mg/day, easily met by average American diet; recommended upper limit to dietary intake of approximately 100 mEq/day (2.4 g/day)

A. Physiologic role of sodium
1. Regulation of fluid distribution in body: water follows sodium; normal extracellular fluid (ECF) concentration of sodium 135–145 mEq/L; normal intracellular fluid (ICF) concentration of sodium 10 mEq/L; 95% of physiologically active sodium is in ECF
2. Maintenance of body fluid osmolality: most abundant cation in ECF; doubling of serum sodium concentration gives approximate serum osmolality
3. Promotion of neuromuscular response: Transmission of nerve and muscle impulses depends on sodium gradient (asymmetric distribution) between ECF and ICF.
    a) Sodium-potassium pump: maintains sodium gradient across cell membrane; maintains voltage action potential
    b) Depolarization: Sodium shifts into cell, and potassium shifts out.
    c) Repolarization: Sodium shifts out of cell, and potassium shifts in.
    d) Depolarization and repolarization sequence: basis of nerve and muscle impulse transmission
    e) Maintenance of sodium gradient: requires both expenditure of cellular energy (ATP) and adequate ECF sodium
4. Regulation of acid-base balance: Sodium combines with chloride and bicarbonate to alter pH. (See Chapter 4 for a complete discussion of acid-base balance.)
5. Normal regulation of sodium levels
    a) Hypothalamus: manufactures antidiuretic hormone (ADH), which increases sodium and water retention in kidney
    b) Posterior pituitary gland (posterior hypophysis): stores ADH and releases it in response to rising serum osmolality
    c) Kidneys: chief regulators; acted on by ADH; site of control of sodium and water excretion/reabsorption is renal tubules
    d) Adrenal cortex of adrenal glands: manufactures aldosterone and cortisol (cortisone); both act to increase sodium absorption from renal tubules; aldosterone much more potent than cortisol

B. Sodium deficit: hyponatremia, decreased serum sodium—serum sodium less than 135 mEq/L; results from either loss of sodium or gain in water; free water intake must exceed free water output
1. Pathophysiology and etiology: many causes, often sign of serious underlying disease

a) Gastrointestinal (GI) disorders: vomiting, diarrhea, drainage from suction or fistulas, bulimia, and excessive tap water enemas

b) Losses from the skin: heavy sweating coupled with plain water intake, burns, and disease (e.g., cystic fibrosis)

c) Hormonal factors: increased ADH and decreased aldosterone and/or cortisol

   (1) Syndrome of inappropriate antidiuretic hormone (SIADH): excess ADH causes abnormal water retention and dilution of serum sodium; increased water resorption in distal renal tubules

      (a) Drugs predisposing to SIADH: intravenous cyclophosphamide, vincristine, chlorpropamide, tolbutamide, carbamazepine, amitriptyline, haloperidol, thioridazine, thiothixene, and nonsteroidal anti-inflammatory drugs

      (b) Tumors: oat-cell carcinoma of lung (most common); tumors of pancreas, duodenum, and brain; leukemia; Hodgkin's disease; and lymphoma

      (c) Central nervous system disorders: subarachnoid hemorrhage, head injury, and encephalitis

      (d) Pulmonary diseases: tuberculosis, pneumonia, acute asthma, atelectasis, emphysema, pneumothorax, and acute respiratory failure

      (e) Other causes: surgical pain, anesthesia, and heavy use of narcotics

   (2) Addison's disease: decreased adrenocortical hormone production related to adrenal cortex insufficiency; decreased aldosterone with increased sodium loss and potassium retention

d) Renal losses: salt-wasting kidney disease (e.g., chronic interstitial nephropathy, medullary cystic disease, polycystic kidney disease) and use of thiazide diuretics

e) Altered cellular function: hypervolemic states (e.g., congestive heart failure, cirrhosis)

f) Dietary factors: chronic low-sodium diet, excessive plain water intake (e.g., psychogenic polydipsia), fad diets, and anorexia nervosa

g) Other factors: excessive administration of parenteral hypo-osmolar fluids, third-space shifts (sodium becomes physiologically unavailable), incorrect administration of oxytocin (see section III,B,2 of Chapter 6), and AIDS

h) Fluid-volume status associated with hyponatremia

   (1) Hyponatremia with fluid volume excess (FVE): ECF increased, sodium level decreased by dilution; can occur with congestive heart failure, cirrhosis of the liver, and nephrotic syndrome

   (2) Hyponatremia with fluid volume deficit (FVD): ECF and sodium level decreased; can occur with vomiting, diarrhea, adrenocortical insufficiency, and salt-losing nephritis

       (3) Hyponatremia with normal fluid volume: can occur with SIADH, in which most excess water moves into cells, leaving ECF at approximately normal level

2. Signs and symptoms: Hyponatremia affects cells of central nervous system, neuromuscular tissue, and smooth muscle of GI tract; symptoms depend on magnitude, cause, and rapidity of onset.

  a) Central nervous system changes: related to swelling of brain cells; headache, vertigo, apprehension, lethargy, confusion, depression, seizures, and coma

  b) Neuromuscular changes: muscle weakness and muscle cramps

  c) GI abnormalities: nausea, vomiting, diarrhea, and abdominal cramps

  d) Integumentary changes: dry, pale skin; dry mucous membranes; wrinkled tongue; and fingerprint edema over sternum

  e) Other changes: tachycardia, orthostatic blood pressure drop (when FVD exists), fainting, and collapsed neck veins

  f) Laboratory tests: Results can be affected by fluid-volume status of client.

    (1) Serum sodium less than 135 mEq/L; plasma osmolality less than 280 mOsm/kg (except in pseudohyponatremia; see Nurse Alert, "Pseudohyponatremia")

    (2) Serum potassium increased

    (3) Low BUN and creatinine in SIADH

    (4) Urinary sodium increased to more than 20 mEq/L in SIADH

    (5) Urinary specific gravity (SG) less than 1.008; except in SIADH when SG greater than 1.012; low urine volume

    (6) Hematocrit above normal when FVD exists

  g) Influence of rapidity of onset on development of signs and symptoms

    (1) Chronic: gradual onset; clients often asymptomatic with serum sodium levels of more than 125 mEq/L; cerebral swelling less marked; produces fatigue

! NURSE ALERT !

Pseudohyponatremia

Pseudohyponatremia occurs when the serum sodium level appears to be low, but there is actually an excess of total body sodium. This can happen either when hypervolemia exists and excess fluids dilute the excess sodium, or when marked hyperlipidemia or marked hypoproteinemia is present, or when sodium is sequestered in a third-space fluid shift.

(2) Acute: rapid onset; neurological symptoms more severe; produces shock; higher mortality with rapid onset; usually due to water overload

3. Treatment and management
   a) Restore sodium balance: in severe cases, parenteral administration of normal saline (0.9% NaCl) or hyperosmolar saline (3% or 5% NaCl; see Nurse Alert, "Administration of Hyperosmolar Saline"); rapid infusion may cause pulmonary edema
   b) Stop sodium loss: Treat underlying cause when possible.
   c) Restore fluid balance: temporary fluid restriction in mild cases of hyponatremia due to SIADH; furosemide to promote water excretion

4. Nursing process
   a) Nursing assessment
      (1) Obtain client history relative to high-risk factors for hyponatremia (e.g., vomiting, diarrhea, eating disorders, low-sodium diet).
      (2) Obtain history of medications, with emphasis on those predisposing to hyponatremia (e.g., diuretics).
      (3) Assess for signs of hyponatremia (e.g., headache, fatigue, muscular weakness).
      (4) Obtain baseline laboratory test values (e.g., serum sodium, serum osmolality, serum potassium, serum chloride, urinary SG).
   b) Nursing diagnoses: Often diagnoses are collaborative and related to underlying disease.
      (1) Altered health maintenance related to GI fluid loss, vomiting, diarrhea, or gastric suction
      (2) Altered urinary output related to SIADH secondary to surgery
      (3) Altered health related to administration of medication (diuretics)

❗ N U R S E *A L E R T* ❗

Administration of Hyperosmolar Saline

Hyperosmolar saline (3% or 5% NaCl) can be dangerous when administered incorrectly. The nurse should follow these steps to ensure safe administration.

- Check serum sodium level before and during administration.
- Administer only in intensive care settings.
- Monitor aggressively for signs of pulmonary edema or worsening neurologic symptoms.
- Be aware that only small volumes of hyperosmolar fluids are needed.
- Use volume-controlled apparatus to administer fluid; monitor flow closely.
- Keep rate of sodium increase to no more than 2 mEq/L/hour to a maximum serum sodium concentration of 125 mEq/L.
- Save urine for measurement of electrolyte content.

      c) Nursing interventions
        (1) Monitor laboratory test results, with emphasis on serum sodium.
        (2) Monitor GI fluid losses.
        (3) Keep accurate fluid intake and output records.
        (4) Monitor for changes in central nervous system symptoms (i.e., confusion, lethargy, muscular twitching, convulsions).
        (5) Check frequently for signs of fluid overload in clients receiving parenteral therapy.
        (6) Encourage high-sodium foods (e.g., beef broth, canned tomato juice) in clients able to eat.
        (7) Restrict water intake when hyponatremia is due to FVE.
        (8) Weigh client daily.

C. Sodium excess: hypernatremia, increased serum sodium—serum sodium greater than 145 mEq/L; most common in infants and the elderly
  1. Pathophysiology and etiology
    a) GI disorders: vomiting and diarrhea when water loss is greater than sodium loss (usually in infants and children)
    b) Hormonal factors
      (1) Cushing's syndrome: excess cortisol production associated with hyperfunction of adrenal cortex
      (2) Overproduction of aldosterone by adrenal cortex
      (3) Excess therapeutic intake of adrenal steroids (e.g., cortisone)
    c) Renal factors: decreased renal function; causes reduced glomerular filtration or inappropriate response to hormones
    d) Dietary factors: increased sodium intake and decreased water intake (water deprivation)
    e) Other factors: heavy sweating without replacement fluids, excessive administration of parenteral hyperosmolar fluids, diabetes insipidus with water intake restriction, increased insensible water loss (e.g., hyperventilation), heatstroke, swallowing of seawater, saline-induced abortions
    f) Fluid-volume status associated with hypernatremia
      (1) Hypernatremia with FVE: sodium gained at a greater rate than water, as with too rapid administration of hyperosmolar sodium solutions
      (2) Hypernatremia with FVD: loss of water greater than loss of sodium; heavy sweating, diarrhea (in infants and children), and poor water intake (in the elderly)
      (3) Hypernatremia associated with near normal fluid volume: increased insensible water loss
  2. Signs and symptoms: Hypernatremia is less common than hyponatremia; it is difficult to separate from underlying disease.

a) Central nervous system changes: restlessness, agitation, disorientation, hallucinations, lethargy when undisturbed, irritability when stimulated, seizures, and coma
b) Neuromuscular changes: tremor, muscle twitching, and hyperreflexia
c) GI abnormalities: nausea; vomiting; dry, swollen tongue; and sticky mucous membranes
d) Integumentary changes: flushed, dry skin
e) Other changes: tachycardia, fever, and marked thirst
f) Laboratory tests: Results can be affected by the fluid-volume status of client.
   (1) Serum sodium greater than 145 mEq/L and serum osmolality greater than 295 mOsm/kg
   (2) Urinary SG greater than 1.015, except with diabetes insipidus when SG less than 1.005
   (3) Urinary sodium greater than 40 mEq/L
   (4) Urinary output greater than 200 ml/hour (diabetes insipidus)
g) Influence of rapidity of onset on development of signs and symptoms
   (1) Chronic onset: brain volume adapts to increased sodium; symptoms less pronounced
   (2) Acute onset: more extreme central nervous system symptoms; higher mortality

3. Treatment and management
a) Restore sodium and water balance: in severe cases, parenteral administration of hypo-osmolar fluids (e.g., 0.45% NaCl solution); too rapid reduction of serum sodium levels results in convulsions and coma due to brain cell swelling
b) Correct underlying cause when possible.

4. Nursing process
a) Nursing assessment
   (1) Obtain client history relative to high-risk factors for hypernatremia (e.g., increased sodium intake, water deprivation, increased adrenocortical hormone production, sodium-retaining drugs).
   (2) Assess for signs of hypernatremia (e.g., nausea, vomiting, signs of FVD).
   (3) Obtain baseline values of laboratory tests (e.g., serum sodium, serum osmolality, urine SG).
b) Nursing diagnoses
   (1) Altered nutrition related to excess intake of sodium-rich foods
   (2) Inadequate fluid replacement related to excess sweating
c) Nursing interventions
   (1) Monitor laboratory test results, with emphasis on serum sodium and serum osmolality.
   (2) Keep accurate fluid intake and output records.
   (3) Monitor for signs of pulmonary edema when client is receiving large amounts of normal saline or any amount of concentrated saline IV.

    (4) Offer assistance in drinking to clients able to take water by mouth.

    (5) Teach client to avoid sodium-rich foods.

    (6) Teach client to avoid heat stress (see Client Teaching Checklist, "Avoiding Heat Stress").

    (7) Weigh client daily.

See text pages

III. Potassium (K) imbalances: common in clinical practice either because of association with underlying disease or injury or induced by medication; dietary requirement 40–60 mEq/day (1.6–2.4 g/day), normally met by balanced diet; potassium not stored well in cells

A. Physiologic role of potassium

    1. Regulation of fluid volume within the cell: 97% of potassium found in ICF, but normal clinical measure is serum potassium because of ease of measurement; normal serum potassium level in adults 3.5–5.0 mEq/L, in children 3.4–4.7 mEq/L, in infants 4.1–5.3 mEq/L; intracellular potassium level (rarely measured) about 150 mEq/L

    2. Promotion of nerve impulse transmission

    3. Contraction of skeletal, smooth, and cardiac muscle

    4. Control of hydrogen ion (H^+) concentration, acid-base balance: When potassium moves out of cell, hydrogen ions move in and vice versa.

    5. Plays a role in enzyme action for cellular energy production

---

✔ CLIENT TEACHING CHECKLIST ✔

Avoiding Heat Stress

Heat stress and accompanying electrolyte imbalances can produce symptoms ranging from mild dizziness to coma and death. Advise the client of the following approaches to preventing heat stress.

✔ Allowing time to acclimate to a hot environment
✔ Gradually increasing over a period of 1–3 weeks heavy work performed in a hot environment
✔ Replacing lost fluids at regular intervals
✔ Replacing lost electrolytes with a commercial electrolyte-rehydrating solution (e.g., Gatorade)
✔ Avoiding strenuous activity during the hottest part of the day
✔ Wearing clothing that allows sweat to evaporate

6. Normal regulation of potassium levels
   a) Sodium-potassium pump: maintains high ICF concentration of potassium
   b) Adrenal cortex of adrenal glands: manufactures aldosterone, which promotes potassium excretion
   c) Kidneys: main regulator; 80%–90% of potassium excreted through kidneys; remainder lost through skin and bowel
      (1) Proximal tubules of kidney always resorb most filtered potassium regardless of intake.
      (2) Distal tubules of kidney regulate potassium excretion/resorption in response to changing serum levels of potassium (aldosterone acts here).

B. Potassium deficit: hypokalemia, hypopotassemia, decreased serum potassium—serum potassium values below 3.5 mEq/L; results from decreased intake or increased loss of potassium
   1. Pathophysiology and etiology: Many diseases and medications predispose to this condition.
      a) GI disorders: most common source of potassium loss; vomiting, diarrhea, gastric or intestinal suctioning or fistula, laxative abuse, bulimia, enema abuse, and disease (e.g., villous adenomas)
      b) Hormonal factors: aldosterone and cortisol promote potassium excretion; Cushing's syndrome and stress (increased adrenocortical hormones)
      c) Renal losses: potassium-wasting diuretics main cause
         (1) Drugs predisposing to renal loss: potassium-wasting diuretics (e.g., thiazides alone or in conjunction with furosemide), corticosteroids (e.g., cortisone, prednisone), levodopa, lithium, antibiotics (e.g., amphotericin, neomycin, cisplatin, ampicillin, carbenicillin, sodium penicillins) alpha-adrenergic blockers, beta$_2$ agonists, estrogen, and laxatives
         (2) Other causes of renal loss: European licorice (contains an agent that mimics action of aldosterone), excess steroid administration (e.g., for asthma), and adrenal adenomas
      d) Dietary factors: malnutrition, starvation, alcoholism, crash diets, and anorexia nervosa; poor intake often coupled with additional predisposing factors
      e) Altered cellular function: trauma, tissue damage, surgery, and burns (potassium needed for new cells)
      f) Redistribution of potassium into cells
         (1) Alkalosis (rising pH): Potassium moves into cells as hydrogen ions move out to correct pH (electroneutrality must be maintained); serum potassium values decrease, but total potassium in body remains the same.
         (2) Insulin: promotes movement of glucose and potassium into cells
   2. Signs and symptoms: widespread derangement of normal physiologic functioning

a) Cardiac abnormalities: can be severe, ending in circulatory failure and systolic arrest
   (1) Atrial and ventricular arrhythmias (dysrhythmias): related to changes in electrophysiology (repolarization) and conductivity; especially severe in clients with ischemic myocardial disease
   (2) Electrocardiogram (ECG/EKG) abnormalities: changes in serial ECGs good indication of direction serum potassium level is moving
      (a) T waves become flat or inverted.
      (b) S-T segment becomes depressed.
      (c) Q-T interval becomes prolonged.
      (d) U wave becomes prominent.
b) GI abnormalities: abdominal distension, decreased peristalsis (silent ileus), nausea, vomiting, diarrhea, and anorexia
c) Neuromuscular changes: muscle weakness, muscle flaccidity, muscle cramps, fatigue, confusion, paresthesia, diminished deep-tendon reflex, and respiratory paralysis
d) Renal changes: polyuria related to decreased responsiveness to ADH
e) Laboratory tests
   (1) Serum potassium <3.5 mEq/L
   (2) Serum osmolality <280 mOsm/L
   (3) Increased pH when alkalosis present
3. Treatment and management: frequently complicated by presence of other disease conditions
   a) Restore potassium balance.
      (1) Oral supplements in the form of potassium chloride, potassium citrate, or potassium gluconate tablets for mild to moderate cases
      (2) Parenteral replacement therapy in the form of potassium chloride, potassium phosphate, or potassium acetate for severe, life-threatening cases; extreme caution needed when giving IV potassium replacement, as cardiac muscle is highly sensitive to ECF potassium; slow administration of correct dilution gives potassium time to enter cells
   b) Prevent hypokalemia: diet of foods rich in potassium (e.g., bananas, orange juice, meat broths)
4. Nursing process
   a) Nursing assessment
      (1) Obtain client history relative to high-risk factors for hypokalemia (e.g., vomiting, renal disease, diuretic use).
      (2) Assess for signs of hypokalemia (e.g., muscle weakness, abdominal distension, decreased peristalsis).

(3) Obtain baseline laboratory test values: ECG reading, serum potassium, and serum osmolality.
b) Nursing diagnoses: usually a collaborative diagnosis because of underlying disease
    (1) Altered nutrition, less than body requirements, related to insufficient intake of potassium-rich foods
    (2) Altered nutrition, less than body requirements, related to high potassium losses (e.g., gastric suctioning)
    (3) Impaired physical mobility relative to potassium deficit
c) Nursing interventions
    (1) Monitor laboratory test results, with special attention to changes in ECG patterns and in serum potassium.
    (2) Keep accurate fluid intake and output records.
    (3) Monitor for changes in cardiac response and other signs of worsening hypokalemia.
    (4) Monitor for signs of phlebitis (potassium irritates veins) when potassium given IV.
    (5) Educate client about eating high-potassium foods.

C. Potassium excess: hyperkalemia, hyperpotassemia, increased serum potassium—serum potassium greater than 5.0 mEq/L in adults; false readings (pseudohyperkalemia) can occur (see Nurse Alert, "Pseudohyperkalemia")
  1. Pathology and etiology: either absolute gain in potassium in body or shift of potassium from ICF to ECF
    a) Renal factors: acute or chronic renal failure, potassium-sparing diuretics; serum potassium increases when urine output is severely decreased (oliguria) or interrupted (anuria)

! **NURSE ALERT** !

Pseudohyperkalemia

Pseudohyperkalemia, or a falsely high serum potassium reading, can result from the way blood is drawn. If blood cells are ruptured in the collection process, potassium is released into the extracellular fluid and gives a falsely elevated reading. To avoid pseudohyperkalemia the nurse should

- Never use a sample when the blood is grossly hemolyzed.
- Never draw blood from an area above the site where potassium is being infused.
- Avoid drawing a sample from an arm that performed repeated fist clenching before the blood is to be drawn.
- Avoid prolonged tight application of a tourniquet before drawing blood.
- Avoid drawing blood with needles having a lumen of less than 18 gauge.

      b) Hormonal factors: Addison's disease; reduced secretion of aldosterone causes retention of potassium.

      c) Altered cellular function: severe traumatic injury, crushing injuries, and burns (cells break down), metabolic acidosis; increased potassium movement into ECF

      d) Excessive potassium intake: overuse of oral potassium supplements or potassium-rich salt substitutes (often in conjunction with poor renal function or potassium-sparing diuretics); excessive IV potassium infusions; and rapid transfusion of aged blood (aged blood has increased potassium level)

      e) Drugs predisposing to hyperkalemia: K penicillin, indomethacin, captopril, heparin, barbiturates, sedatives, narcotics, amphetamines, nonsteroidal anti-inflammatory drugs (e.g., ibuprofen), alpha agonists, beta blockers, succinylcholine, cyclophosphamide, and potassium-sparing diuretics

      f) Other causes: hyperglycemia with insulin deficiency; severe digitalis toxicity (sodium-potassium pump is poisoned)

  2. Signs and symptoms

    a) Cardiac changes

      (1) Tachycardia followed by bradycardia followed by cardiac arrest (severe hyperkalemia)

      (2) ECG abnormalities

        (a) Peaked, narrow T waves

        (b) Q-T interval shortened

        (c) P-R interval prolonged followed by disappearance of P wave

        (d) QRS interval prolonged

    b) GI abnormalities: abdominal cramps, nausea, and diarrhea

    c) Neuromuscular changes: muscle weakness, paresthesia, and muscle cramps; client remains alert

    d) Laboratory tests: serum potassium greater than 5.0 mEq/L, often pH decreased (acidosis)

  3. Treatment and management

    a) Restrict potassium intake: for mild hyperkalemia; dietary restrictions, discontinue drugs predisposing to hyperkalemia

    b) Remove potassium: sodium polystyrene sulfonate resin (Kayexalate) given orally or rectally exchanges potassium for sodium ions; dialysis used in critical situations

    c) Take emergency stopgap measures: buy time; either IV administration of sodium bicarbonate or insulin with glucose (moves potassium back into cells) or IV administration of 10% calcium gluconate (decreases irritability of myocardium); no potassium removal: not permanent solution

4. Nursing process
   a) Nursing assessment
      (1) Obtain client history relative to high-risk factors for hyperkalemia (e.g., renal disease, potassium-sparing diuretics, excessive salt substitute use).
      (2) Assess for signs of hyperkalemia (e.g., cardiac arrhythmia).
      (3) Obtain baseline ECG; assess for altered T waves.
      (4) Obtain baseline value for serum potassium.
   b) Nursing diagnoses
      (1) High risk for decreased cardiac output related to arrhythmia secondary to hyperkalemia
      (2) Altered urinary elimination related to renal dysfunction
   c) Nursing interventions
      (1) Monitor vital signs, with special attention to tachycardia and bradycardia.
      (2) Monitor changes in ECG patterns, with special attention to peaked T waves, wide QRS complex, and prolonged P-R interval.
      (3) Monitor serum potassium level.
      (4) Keep accurate fluid intake and output records.
      (5) Educate client concerning use of salt substitutes, potassium-sparing diuretics, and other predisposing drugs.

IV. Calcium (Ca) imbalances: many causes because calcium is regulated by many factors; often a medical emergency because of calcium's effects on heart muscle; minimum daily requirement 800 mg/day (higher in adolescents, young adults, pregnant and lactating women, postmenopausal women, and adults older than age 65)

See text pages
_____

A. Physiologic role of calcium
   1. Distribution of calcium in the body
      a) 99% of calcium found in bones and teeth; physiologically unavailable
      b) 1% calcium in ECF; serum calcium (total serum calcium); normal level 4.5–5.5 mEq/L (9–11 mg/dl)
      c) More than half of calcium in ECF bound to protein, mainly albumin; cannot cross capillary membranes to leave vascular system; accounts for about 53% of serum calcium
      d) Ionized calcium (iCa) physiologically active, crosses cell membranes; accounts for 47% serum calcium; normal value 2.2–2.5 mEq/L (4.5–5.0 mg/dl)
   2. Maintenance of skeletal elements: calcium needed for strong, durable bones and teeth; exchanges only very slowly with serum calcium
   3. Regulation of neuromuscular activity: ionized calcium
      a) Regulates cell membrane permeability: Increased calcium decreases permeability.
      b) Regulates transmission of nerve impulse: nerve cells less excitable when adequate calcium is present

      c) Regulates muscle contraction and relaxation: vital in regulation of heartbeat

    4. Influence on enzyme activity: ionized calcium; activates many enzymes vital to body function

    5. Other roles: functions in blood coagulation by converting prothrombin to thrombin; necessary part of material that holds cells together

    6. Normal regulation of calcium levels: bone resorption, renal resorption, and intestinal absorption

      a) Parathyroid hormone (PTH): secreted by parathyroid glands embedded in thyroid; promotes transfer of calcium from bone to plasma, raising serum calcium level; promotes absorption of calcium from small intestine; enhances renal absorption of calcium; secreted in response to low serum calcium

      b) Calcitonin (thyrocalcitonin): hormone produced by thyroid gland; effects opposite those of PTH; promotes transfer of calcium from plasma to bone, lowering serum calcium level; secreted in response to high serum calcium

      c) Vitamin D: ingested in food or synthesized in body; most active form is called calcitriol; increases calcium absorption from intestine and aids PTH in mobilizing bone calcium; enhances calcium and phosphorus available for new bone formation

B. Calcium deficit: hypocalcemia—serum calcium less than 4.5 mEq/L

    1. Pathophysiology and etiology: results from inadequate intake or decreased absorption from intestine

      a) Dietary factors: inadequate calcium in food; lack of vitamin D (needed for calcium absorption); inadequate protein in diet (inhibits body's use of calcium)

      b) GI factors: decreased absorption due to pancreatitis, Crohn's disease, resection of small bowel, or chronic diarrhea

      c) Hormonal factors: PTH deficiency (main cause), often secondary to sepsis, burns, or surgery (e.g., parathyroidectomy, thyroidectomy, radical neck dissection); vitamin D deficiency (may be related to renal failure)

      d) Other electrolyte imbalances: magnesium deficiency of less than 1 mg/dl; increased serum phosphorus, often due to renal failure (as serum phosphorus increases, serum calcium decreases); alkalosis resulting in increased protein-bound calcium, with less ionized calcium available even when total serum calcium is normal; increased serum albumin resulting in increase in bound calcium; rapid dilution of plasma with calcium-free solution

e) Drugs predisposing to hypocalcemia
   (1) Drugs inhibiting PTH secretion: magnesium sulfate, propylthiouracil, colchicine, plicamycin, neomycin, and excessive sodium citrate
   (2) Drugs altering vitamin D metabolism: acetazolamide, aspirin, anticonvulsants (e.g., phenobarbital), glutethimide, estrogens, and aminoglycosides
   (3) Drugs increasing serum phosphate levels: oral, enema, or intravenous sodium phosphate or potassium phosphate
   (4) Drugs decreasing calcium mobilization from bone: corticosteroids (e.g., cortisone, prednisone)
   (5) Drugs decreasing calcium absorption in renal tubules: loop diuretics (e.g., furosemide)
 f) Other causes: alcoholism, medullary thyroid carcinoma, and rapid infusion of banked blood during transfusion (citrate—used as preservative and anticoagulant—binds with ionized calcium)
2. Signs and symptoms: vary widely from client to client based on severity, duration, and rapidity of onset; when hypokalemia present, symptoms are potentiated
 a) Neuromuscular signs: tetany, including neural excitability; tingling and muscle spasms of mouth, hands, and feet; and larynx (severe hypocalcemia)
   (1) Trousseau's sign: A blood pressure cuff inflated at 10–20 mm Hg above systolic pressure on the upper arm

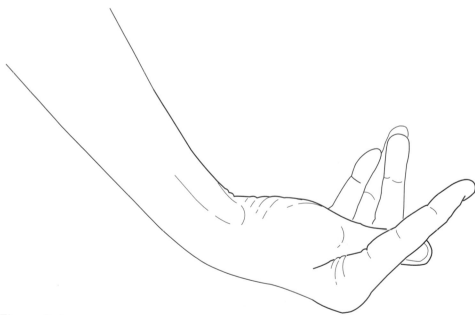

Figure 3–1
Trousseau's Sign

constricts circulation and elicits a carpopedal spasm of the fingers and hands within 1–5 minutes.

(2) Chvostek's sign: The face is tapped over the facial nerve—about 2 cm in front of the earlobe—and elicits facial muscle twitching.

b) Central nervous system changes: irritability, anxiety, delusions, hallucinations, memory impairment, depression, and convulsions

c) Cardiovascular changes

(1) Gross changes: weak cardiac contractions, potential for congestive heart failure

(2) ECG abnormalities

(a) S-T segment lengthened

(b) Q-T interval prolonged

d) Changes in laboratory test values

(1) Serum calcium decreased: except in alkalosis, when serum calcium remains the same but ionized (available) calcium

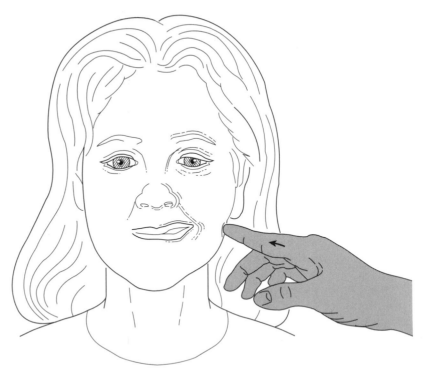

Figure 3–2
Chvostek's Sign

decreases; if serum albumin also low, low serum calcium value may not indicate hypocalcemia

    (2) Ionized calcium decreased: more accurate measurement than serum calcium

    (3) Blood-clotting time increased

  e) Chronic hypocalcemia: osteoporosis (loss of bone mass); due to prolonged low calcium intake; serum calcium levels normal, but total body calcium decreased; increased incidence of skeletal fractures; most at risk are postmenopausal women not taking estrogen replacement therapy, elderly women, and elderly men

3. Treatment and management: Goal is to alleviate underlying cause.

  a) Emergency measures: administration of parenteral calcium salts (e.g., calcium gluconate, calcium chloride, calcium gluceptate diluted with 5% dextrose in water); too rapid administration causes cardiac arrest

  b) Mild or chronic hypocalcemia: foods high in calcium (e.g., milk and milk products, salmon canned with bones), oral calcium supplements, vitamin D supplements, and increased protein in diet

4. Nursing process

  a) Nursing assessment

    (1) Obtain client history relative to potential causes of hypocalcemia (e.g., low-calcium diet, lack of vitamin D, low-protein diet, chronic diarrhea, hormonal disorders).

    (2) Obtain client history relative to drugs predisposing to hypocalcemia (e.g., furosemide, cortisone).

    (3) Assess for signs of hypocalcemia (e.g., tetany symptoms, Trousseau's sign, Chvostek's sign).

    (4) Obtain baseline values for serum calcium, ionized calcium, serum albumin, and acid-base status.

    (5) Obtain baseline ECG, noting abnormalities in S-T segment and Q-T interval.

    (6) Take safety precautions if client is confused or hallucinating.

    (7) Prepare to adopt seizure precautions if hypocalcemia is severe.

  b) Nursing diagnoses

    (1) Altered nutrition related to inadequate intake of calcium, vitamin D, or protein

    (2) Altered nutrition relative to inadequate calcium absorption

    (3) High risk for injury, bleeding, related to interference with coagulation secondary to calcium loss

  c) Nursing interventions

    (1) Monitor laboratory test results, with emphasis on serum and ionized calcium.

    (2) Monitor ECGs for changes in pattern.

    (3) When calcium is given parenterally, monitor for irritation of subcutaneous tissue and tissue sloughing.

    (4) Teach client to eat high-calcium foods; educate client concerning prevention of osteoporosis.

            (5) Educate client concerning proper, moderate use of laxatives and antacids.

            (6) Monitor for signs of cardiac arrhythmias in clients receiving digitalis and calcium supplements (either oral or IV).

            (7) Monitor for hypocalcemia in clients receiving massive transfusions of citrated blood.

C. Calcium excess: hypercalcemia—serum calcium greater than 5.5 mEq/L (11 mg/dl)

   1. Pathophysiology and etiology: excessive release of bone calcium, almost always from malignancy; hyperparathyroidism; thiazide-diuretic use; excessive calcium intake; excessive vitamin D

     a) Malignancy: 25%–50% of malignancies in lung, breast, ovaries, prostate, and bladder cause hypercalcemia.

       (1) Bone metastasis increases bone breakdown and resorption; kidneys unable to excrete calcium fast enough, so serum level rises

       (2) Parathyroid hormone that is produced ectopically by tumors releases calcium from bone; GI and renal absorption increased

     b) Dietary factors: increased calcium intake through supplements or heavy antacid use (often coupled with high milk intake as in peptic ulcer)

     c) Hormonal influences: primary parahyperthyroidism (e.g., benign adenoma); same actions as ectopic PTH production

     d) Drugs predisposing to hypercalcemia: calcium salts (oral or IV supplements), megadoses of vitamin A or D, thiazide diuretics (potentiate action of PTH), androgens or estrogens for breast cancer therapy, IV lipids, lithium, and tamoxifen

     e) Prolonged immobilization: causes resorption of bone; most conspicuous in adolescents and those with Paget's disease

   2. Signs and symptoms: magnitude of elevation and rapidity of onset affect symptoms: acute hypercalcemia more symptomatic than chronic condition

     a) Neuromuscular changes: decreased neuromuscular excitability, muscle weakness, muscle flaccidity, and depressed deep-tendon reflex

     b) GI changes: constipation from decreased smooth muscle motility, delayed gastric emptying, anorexia, nausea, and vomiting; clients also predisposed to duodenal ulcer (10%–20%) or pancreatitis (35%)

     c) Central nervous system changes: depression and apathy; with severe elevations, memory loss and acute psychosis

     d) Renal changes: polyuria, formation of kidney stones (renal calculi) from excess calcium; with severe elevation, acute and nonreversible renal failure

    e) Cardiovascular changes
       (1) Gross changes: bradycardia, increased contractility, and ventricular arrhythmias
       (2) ECG abnormalities
         (a) Q-T interval shortens; T waves invert
         (b) S-T segment shortens or diminishes
    f) Other changes: deep bone pain; radiographic evidence of bone thinning

3. Treatment and management: immediate reduction of serum calcium and correction of underlying cause
    a) Increase urinary calcium excretion: IV normal saline given with furosemide; oral or retention enema phosphate salts (risk of soft tissue calcification); calcitonin; intravenous phosphates (high-risk, hypercalcemic crisis only)
    b) Inhibit resorption from bone: Plicamycin (antitumor antibiotic) inhibits action of PTH on osteoblasts (bone cells); calcitonin inhibits effects of PTH; diphosphonates (oral or IV) retard bone turnover.
    c) Decrease intestinal calcium resorption: Glucocorticoids (e.g., cortisone) compete with vitamin D, decreasing intestinal absorption.
    d) Eliminate drugs predisposing to hypercalcemia.
    e) Initiate peritoneal dialysis or hemodialysis only for hypercalcemic crisis when other measures fail.

4. Nursing process
    a) Nursing assessment
       (1) Obtain client history to identify probable cause of hypercalcemia (e.g., cancer; excessive use of calcium supplements, antacids, or thiazide diuretics; steroid therapy).
       (2) Assess for signs of hypercalcemia (e.g., deep bone pain, flaccid muscles, kidney stones).
       (3) Obtain baseline values for serum calcium and serum phosphate.
       (4) Obtain baseline ECG, noting any abnormalities in Q-T interval or S-T segment.
       (5) Assess client's fluid volume status and mental alertness.
    b) Nursing diagnoses: Many collaborative diagnoses are related to underlying cause (e.g., cancers).
       (1) Altered nutrition, more than body requirement, related to excess calcium intake
       (2) High risk for injury related to bone destruction due to cancer
       (3) Altered pattern of urinary elimination related to causes of hypercalcemia
    c) Nursing interventions
       (1) Monitor changes in vital signs, laboratory test results, and ECGs.
       (2) Encourage client to drink 3–4 liters of fluids per day, including sodium-containing fluids unless contraindicated, to help prevent formation of renal calculi.

(3) Encourage client to consume fluids (e.g., cranberry or prune juice) that promote urine acidity to help prevent formation of renal calculi.
(4) Keep accurate fluid intake and output records.
(5) Monitor for digitalis toxicity.
(6) Handle client gently to prevent fractures.
(7) Encourage passive exercise for bedridden clients.
(8) Educate client to avoid high-calcium foods (e.g., milk products).
(9) Educate clients with cancers (and those clients' families) about symptoms of hypercalcemia.

See text pages

V. Magnesium (Mg) imbalances: minimum daily adult requirement 280–350 mg/day (higher in adolescents and lactating women)

A. Physiologic role of magnesium: second-most-plentiful cation in ICF (after potassium)
  1. Distribution of magnesium in the body
    a) 67% contained in bone; physiologically unavailable
    b) 31% contained in ICF
    c) 1% contained in ECF: normal adult serum magnesium level 1.3–2.1 mEq/L (1.6–2.5 mg/dl); lower in infants; 67% ionized, 33% bound to protein
    d) Lower GI tract: 10–14 mEq/L compared with 1–2 mEq/L of upper GI tract
    e) Cerebrospinal fluid: concentration higher than in blood
  2. Enzyme activation: needed for B vitamins and enzymes associated with carbohydrate and protein metabolism to function; required for synthesis of nucleic acids
  3. Regulation of neuromuscular activity: similar to calcium
    a) Regulates skeletal and heart muscle contractions: depresses acetylcholine release at synaptic junction
    b) Mediates transmission of nerve impulses: Neuromuscular activity increases as magnesium levels decrease.
  4. Regulation of electrolyte balance
    a) Facilitates transportation of sodium and potassium across cell membranes
    b) Influences intracellular calcium through effect on PTH; low magnesium levels impair action of PTH
    c) Influences utilization of calcium, potassium, and protein
  5. Normal regulation of magnesium
    a) Diet: Sources include green vegetables, whole seeds and grains, nuts (e.g., peanut butter), legumes, bananas, grapefruit, and chocolate.

b) Absorption from the intestine: influenced by length of time in intestine, rate of water absorption, and amounts of calcium, phosphate, and lactose in diet

c) Kidneys: resorbed primarily in loop of Henle of kidney; magnesium conserving, may excrete as little as 1 mEq/day when body levels are low

B. Magnesium deficit: hypomagnesemia—serum level less than 1.3 mEq/L; 40% of clients also have hypokalemia; also found in conjunction with hypocalcemia

1. Pathophysiology and etiology: common in critically ill clients, but frequently undiagnosed; client often remains asymptomatic until serum level reaches 1.0 mEq/L

   a) GI losses

      (1) Distal small bowel: site of most magnesium resorption; disrupted by chronic diarrhea, prolonged laxative use, malabsorption syndromes (e.g., nontropical sprue, steatorrhea), small bowel resection, and inflammatory bowel disease

      (2) Drainage from intestinal fistulas

      (3) Nasogastric suction in conjunction with use of magnesium-free parenteral fluids

   b) Renal losses: excessive renal excretion due to potassium-wasting diuretic use; diuresis due to diabetic ketoacidosis and high glucose load

   c) Chronic alcoholism: most common cause in United States; due to decreased magnesium intake and accelerated GI losses

   d) Dietary factors: malnutrition, starvation, and total parenteral nutrition (TPN) without magnesium supplements

   e) Drugs predisposing toward hypomagnesemia: potassium-wasting (loop) diuretics (e.g., furosemide, bumetanide, ethacrynic acid), aminoglycosides (e.g., gentamicin, tobramycin, kanamycin), cortisone, amphotericin, digitalis (hypomagnesemia promotes digitalis toxicity), cisplatin, and cyclosporin

   f) Other causes: rapid administration of citrated blood, increased calcium intake, and major surgery

2. Signs and symptoms: Hypomagnesemia can cause hypocalcemia or hypokalemia or both.

   a) Neuromuscular changes: Main symptoms are neuromuscular.

      (1) Muscle weakness with hyperexcitability, tremor, athetoid and choreiform movements (slow, involuntary writhing and twisting), paresthesia, convulsions

      (2) Positive Trousseau's sign (see this chapter, section IV,B,2,a,1)

      (3) Positive Chvostek's sign (see this chapter, section IV,B,2,a,2)

   b) Central nervous system changes: agitation, depression, personality changes, confusion, and auditory and visual hallucinations

   c) Cardiovascular abnormalities

      (1) Gross changes: arrhythmias (e.g., premature ventricular contractions, ventricular tachycardia, ventricular fibrillation)

  (2) ECG abnormalities
    (a) P-R and Q-T intervals are prolonged.
    (b) QRS complex widens.
    (c) T wave becomes flat or inverted.
    (d) S-T segment is depressed.
  d) Laboratory test values: often test not ordered in standard clinical blood work
3. Treatment and management: Hypokalemia that does not respond to potassium replacement often indicates hypomagnesemia.
  a) Mild hypomagnesemia: increase client's intake of green vegetables, whole grains and seeds, nuts, and legumes; oral magnesium salts (e.g., magnesium sulfate, magnesium citrate); side effect diarrhea
  b) Severe hypomagnesemia: repeated deep intramuscular injections of magnesium salts; IV magnesium sulfate; requires extreme caution (see this chapter, section V,B,4,c,5)
4. Nursing process
  a) Nursing assessment
    (1) Obtain client history, being especially alert to factors predisposing to hypomagnesemia (e.g., alcoholism, laxative abuse, TPN, potassium-wasting diuretic use).
    (2) Assess for signs and symptoms of hypomagnesemia (e.g., tetany, tremors, twitches, cardiac arrhythmias).
    (3) Obtain baseline values for laboratory tests: serum magnesium, serum calcium, and serum potassium.
    (4) Obtain baseline ECG, noting abnormalities in P-R and Q-T intervals, QRS complex, T wave, and S-T segment.
  b) Nursing diagnoses: Clients with hypomagnesemia are often critically ill with other electrolyte imbalances.
    (1) Altered nutrition, less than body requirements, related to chronic alcoholism, chronic laxative abuse, chronic diarrhea, or poor nutritional intake
    (2) High risk for injury related to serum magnesium deficit
    (3) Decreased cardiac output related to serum magnesium deficit
  c) Nursing interventions
    (1) Monitor vital signs, changes in ECGs, and changes in laboratory test values.
    (2) Closely monitor for digitalis toxicity (e.g., nausea, vomiting, bradycardia) those clients taking digitalis.
    (3) Keep accurate fluid intake and output records.
    (4) Take safety precautions if client is mentally confused.
    (5) Administer magnesium replacement therapy as directed by physician; monitor continuously for abatement of symptoms

of hypomagnesemia and appearance of symptoms of hypermagnesemia those clients receiving IV therapy.

    (6) Educate clients about appropriate use of laxatives or diuretics if deficit is due to abuse.

    (7) Encourage clients able to eat a general diet to consume foods high in magnesium.

C. Magnesium excess: hypermagnesemia—serum level greater than 2.1 mEq/L; relatively rare

  1. Pathophysiology and etiology

    a) Renal factors: advanced renal failure; inadequate excretion of magnesium by kidneys (most common cause); greatest risk when age-related, reduced renal function is coupled with magnesium-containing antacid and laxative use

    b) Other causes: severe dehydration from diabetic ketoacidosis; overly aggressive treatment with magnesium salts (sometimes given to delay delivery or treat eclampsia, i.e., convulsions or coma during pregnancy or immediately after delivery)

    c) Drugs predisposing to hypermagnesemia: either lithium or excess use of magnesium salts (e.g., magnesium sulfate, magnesium hydroxide)

  2. Signs and symptoms

    a) GI: nausea and vomiting

    b) Neuromuscular changes (listed from mild to severe): drowsiness, decreased deep-tendon reflex, muscle weakness, loss of patellar reflex (knee jerk), respiratory depression, respiratory paralysis, and coma

    c) Cardiovascular abnormalities (listed from mild to severe): peripheral vasodilation, flushing, sense of warmth, hypotension gradually becoming more pronounced, and cardiac arrest

    d) Electrocardiograph abnormalities

      (1) QRS complex widens.

      (2) P-R and Q-T intervals become prolonged.

  3. Treatment and management: Best treatment is prevention.

    a) Reduce magnesium level: Discontinue parenteral or oral magnesium salts; administer IV calcium (a direct antagonist to magnesium), IV saline, or hemodialysis; provide ventilatory assistance if respiration is impaired.

    b) Correct underlying cause when possible.

  4. Nursing process

    a) Nursing assessment

      (1) Assess for possible causes of hypermagnesemia (e.g., renal insufficiency, chronic laxative use).

      (2) Assess for signs of hypermagnesemia (e.g., drowsiness, hypotension, decreased respiration, periods of apnea)

      (3) Obtain baseline values for serum magnesium, serum calcium, and other electrolytes.

      (4) Obtain baseline ECG, noting any abnormalities in QRS complex, P-R interval, or Q-T interval.

      b) Nursing diagnoses

         (1) Altered nutrition, more than body requirements, related to excess oral or intravenous magnesium administration

         (2) Altered urinary output, less than normal, related to acute renal failure

      c) Nursing interventions

         (1) Monitor vital signs: Clients receiving IV calcium must be monitored continuously.

         (2) Monitor laboratory test values, reporting significant changes.

         (3) Monitor ECGs, noting changes in QRS complex, P-R interval, and Q-T interval.

         (4) Educate clients with renal insufficiencies as to magnesium content of common over-the-counter laxatives and antacids.

         (5) Encourage fluid intake in clients if not contraindicated.

         (6) Be prepared to provide ventilatory assistance or resuscitation.

See text pages
_____

VI. Phosphorus (P) imbalances: major intracellular anion; requirement for adults 800 mg/day; major dietary sources include milk, meat, poultry, fish, grains, dried beans, and legumes

A. Physiologic role of phosphorus: essential to all cells; normal adult serum phosphate level 1.7–2.6 mEq/L (2.5–4.5 mg/dl), higher in children due to greater skeletal muscle growth

    1. Distribution of phosphorus in the body

      a) 85% in bones

      b) Most of the remaining 15% in ICF

    2. Intermediary in metabolism: functions in metabolism of proteins, carbohydrates, and fat

    3. Essential to energy: necessary in formation of high-energy compounds ATP (adenosine triphosphate) and ADP (adenosine diphosphate)

    4. Cellular building block: backbone of nucleic acids, essential to cell membrane formation

    5. Delivery of oxygen: functions in formation of red-blood-cell enzyme 2,3-diphosphoglycerate (2,3-DPG) responsible for oxygen delivery to cells

    6. Acid-base buffer

    7. Normal regulation of phosphorus: low serum phosphate levels stimulate kidney to provide calcitriol, which increases phosphorus absorption from small intestine and resorption by the kidney; when serum phosphate levels are high, PTH overrides calcitriol and stimulates excretion by renal tubules; 90% of phosphorus excreted by kidneys; 10% excreted by GI tract (e.g., in feces)

B. Phosphorus deficit: hypophosphatemia—serum phosphate level below 1.7 mEq/L (2.5 mg/dl)

1. Pathophysiology and etiology
   a) Dietary factors: malnutrition followed by overzealous refeeding, TPN without adequate phosphorus replacement; phosphorus shifts into cells, leaving serum deficit
   b) GI losses: vomiting, anorexia, chronic diarrhea, or malabsorption syndrome (interferes with absorption from jejunum)
   c) Chronic alcoholism: promotes dietary imbalances and diuresis; affects up to 50% of clients hospitalized with this condition
   d) Hormonal influences: hyperparathyroidism; enhances renal phosphate excretion
   e) Acid-base balance: respiratory alkalosis and hyperventilation; shifts phosphorus into cells, lowering serum level
   f) Drugs predisposing to hypophosphatemia: aluminum-containing antacids (e.g., Maalox, Gelusil, Mylanta) bind phosphorus, thereby lowering serum levels; diuretics (e.g., thiazide, acetazolamide) increase renal excretion; androgens, corticosteroids, glucagon, epinephrine, gastrin, and mannitol
   g) Other causes: diabetic ketoacidosis; increased glycogen and polyuria increase renal excretion; dextrose with insulin causes shift of phosphorus into cells; burns cause increased demand in tissue rebuilding
2. Signs and symptoms: often very vague; most result from deficiency of ATP or 2,3-DPG or both
   a) Neurologic changes: weakness, irritability, numbness, paresthesia, confusion, convulsions, and coma
   b) Hemodynamic changes: reduced oxygen delivery to cells (tissue hypoxia), possible increased clotting time (platelet dysfunction), and possible infection (leukocyte dysfunction)
   c) Cardiopulmonary changes: weak pulse and hyperventilation
3. Treatment and management
   a) Mild to moderate: Improve client's nutrition; increase intake of foods high in phosphorus (e.g., skim milk, beef, pork, whole grains, dried beans)
   b) Severe: oral replacement with sodium phosphate (e.g., Phospho-Soda) or potassium phosphate (e.g., Neutra-Phos K); IV replacement with former if serum levels fall below 1 mg/dl
4. Nursing process
   a) Nursing assessment
      (1) Obtain client history, being especially alert to identify factors that put clients at high risk for hypophosphatemia (e.g., alcoholism, TPN, diabetic ketoacidosis).
      (2) Assess for signs of hypophosphatemia (e.g., muscle weakness, hyperventilation, confusion).
      (3) Obtain baseline values for laboratory tests for serum phosphate, serum calcium, and other electrolytes.
   b) Nursing diagnoses
      (1) Altered nutrition, less than body requirements, related to inadequate phosphorus intake, lack of vitamin D, or TPN without phosphorus replacement

    (2) Altered nutrition, less than body requirements, related to inadequate nutrient absorption secondary to chronic diarrhea or chronic alcoholism

   c) Nursing interventions

    (1) Monitor for cardiac, GI, and neurologic abnormalities related to decreased phosphorus level.

    (2) Monitor changes in laboratory test values, with emphasis on serum phosphate and serum calcium.

    (3) Keep accurate records of fluid intake and output.

    (4) Take safety precautions when client is confused.

    (5) Be alert to signs of hypophosphatemia when feeding is restarted after prolonged starvation (refeeding syndrome).

    (6) Be alert to complications of IV administration of phosphorus (e.g., hypocalcemia, hyperphosphatemia).

    (7) Educate client to avoid antacids containing aluminum hydroxide (e.g., Amphojel) to reduce phosphorus binding.

    (8) Educate client concerning consumption of high-phosphorus foods (e.g., skim milk).

 C. Phosphorus excess: hyperphosphatemia—serum phosphate levels greater than 2.6 mEq/L (4.5 mg/dl)

  1. Pathophysiology and etiology: Often, cause remains unclear.

   a) Renal factors: renal disease, acute and chronic renal failure; excretion of phosphorus decreased

   b) Chemotherapy: phosphorus released as the result of cell destruction

   c) Hormonal factors: hypoparathyroidism; decreased PTH results in calcium loss and phosphorus excess

   d) Dietary changes: increased intake of oral phosphate supplements or intravenous phosphate; infants fed cow's milk

   e) Drugs predisposing to hyperphosphatemia: oral phosphates, intravenous phosphates, phosphate laxatives, excessive vitamin D, tetracyclines, and methicillin

   f) Other causes: massive blood transfusions (phosphate leaks from blood cells)

  2. Signs and symptoms

   a) Neuromuscular changes: tetany (especially with hypocalcemia), hyperreflexia, flaccid paralysis, and muscle weakness

   b) Cardiovascular abnormality: tachycardia

   c) Soft tissue changes: calcification; precipitation of calcium phosphate in kidney, joints, arteries, skin, and cornea; most prominent in clients with chronic renal failure

   d) Oxygen delivery change: increase in 2,3-DPG

3. Treatment and management
    a) Eliminate source of excess phosphorus (e.g., oral or IV phosphate salts).
    b) Administer phosphate-binding agent (e.g., aluminum hydroxide [Amphojel], aluminum carbonate [Basaljel]).
    c) Alleviate underlying cause.
4. Nursing process
    a) Nursing assessment
        (1) Obtain client history, with emphasis on factors predisposing to hyperphosphatemia (e.g., renal insufficiency, laxative use).
        (2) Assess for signs and symptoms of hyperphosphatemia and concurrent hypocalcemia (e.g., tetany, muscle cramps).
        (3) Obtain baseline laboratory values for serum phosphate, serum calcium, and other electrolytes.
        (4) Check urinary output; less than 600 ml/day increases serum phosphate level.
    b) Nursing diagnoses: altered nutrition, more than body requirements, related to excess intake of phosphate-containing laxatives, oral phosphate salts, or intravenous phosphate salts
    c) Nursing interventions
        (1) Monitor for cardiac, GI, and neuromuscular abnormalities related to increased phosphorus level.
        (2) Monitor changes in laboratory test values, with emphasis on serum phosphate and serum calcium.
        (3) Keep accurate records of fluid intake and output.
        (4) Observe client for signs and symptoms of hypocalcemia (e.g., tetany); when phosphate levels rise, calcium levels fall.
        (5) Educate client concerning high phosphorus content of processed foods, carbonated beverages, and over-the-counter medications.
        (6) Educate client concerning consumption of low-phosphorus foods (e.g., vegetables).

VII. Chloride (Cl) imbalances: anion that usually appears in conjunction with sodium; highest concentration in ECF; estimated minimum adult requirement 750 mg/day, recommended upper limit to dietary intake 100 mEq/day (3.7 g/day)

See text pages

A. Physiologic role of chloride
    1. Distribution of chloride in the body: primarily extracellular, normal serum concentration of chloride 95–108 mEq/L; intracellular concentration only 1 mEq/L
    2. Regulation of serum osmolality: When osmolality increases, both sodium and chloride increase in proportion to water.
    3. Regulation of fluid balance: When sodium is retained, chloride is also retained, causing water retention and increased fluid volume.
    4. Control of acidity of gastric juice: Chloride combines with hydrogen ions in the stomach to form hydrochloric acid (HCl).

5. Regulation of acid-base balance: Along with bicarbonate and sodium, chloride is one of the electrolytes whose excretion/absorption rate varies to maintain normal pH of blood.
6. Role in oxygen–carbon dioxide exchange (chloride shift): When cells are oxygenated, chloride moves from red blood cells into plasma and bicarbonate moves from plasma into blood cells; chloride helps maintain equilibrium and blood pH.
7. Normal regulation of chloride in the body: In renal tubules, for every sodium cation resorbed by the renal tubules, either a chloride or a bicarbonate ion is resorbed; chloride resorption can differ from sodium resorption.

B. Chloride deficit: hypochloremia—serum chloride levels less than 95 mEq/L
   1. Pathophysiology and etiology: Chloride deficiency and potassium deficiency often occur together.
      a) GI abnormalities
         (1) Continuous vomiting and gastric suction; chloride lost as HCl of gastric juice
         (2) Diarrhea: chloride lost through salty GI secretions; chloride and potassium lost together
      b) Renal abnormalities: Prolonged use of diuretics interferes with absorption of chloride ions from renal tubules.
      c) Skin losses: Chloride combined with sodium is lost through excessive sweating due to high environmental temperatures, muscular exercise, or fever.
      d) Dietary changes: Low-sodium diet can result in chloride deficit, as most chloride enters body as salt (NaCl).
      e) Acid-base changes: metabolic alkalosis; as bicarbonate ions increase, chloride ions decrease
      f) Other causes: prolonged use of IV 5% dextrose in water; dilutes serum electrolytes
   2. Signs and symptoms
      a) Neuromuscular abnormalities: hyperexcitability of muscles; tetany, tremors, and twitching
      b) Respiratory changes: slow, shallow breathing
      c) Cardiac abnormalities: decrease in blood pressure with severe chloride deficit and dehydration
   3. Treatment and management
      a) When hypochloremia is accompanied by hypokalemia, both deficiencies must be corrected simultaneously.
      b) Hypochloremia usually indicates alkalosis (hypochloremic alkalosis) resulting from increased bicarbonate.

c) Administration of 5% dextrose in normal saline can be used to help alleviate hypochloremia resulting from IV dilution effects.
4. Nursing process
   a) Nursing assessment
      (1) Obtain client history relative to conditions predisposing to hypochloremia (e.g., continuous vomiting).
      (2) Assess for signs and symptoms of hypochloremia (e.g., tremors, slow and shallow respiration).
      (3) Assess for signs of metabolic alkalosis.
      (4) Obtain baseline laboratory test values for serum chloride.
   b) Nursing diagnoses: altered health maintenance related to dietary changes, GI abnormalities, or acid-base imbalance
   c) Nursing interventions
      (1) Monitor changes in laboratory test values, with emphasis on serum chloride and serum potassium.
      (2) Monitor for worsening signs of hypochloremia (e.g., drop in blood pressure).
      (3) Monitor serum carbon dioxide or arterial bicarbonate for metabolic alkalosis.
      (4) Keep an accurate record of gastric secretions lost from the body.

C. Chloride excess: hyperchloremia—serum chloride levels greater than 108 mEq/L
   1. Pathophysiology and etiology
      a) Body fluid losses: Severe dehydration elevates serum electrolytes, including chlorides.
      b) Hormonal factors: Excessive adrenal cortical hormone causes a sodium excess and, secondarily, a chloride excess.
      c) Trauma: head injury; sodium and chloride retained
      d) Acid-base imbalance: metabolic acidosis; as bicarbonate ions decrease, chloride ions increase
   2. Signs and symptoms
      a) Neuromuscular changes: weakness and lethargy leading to coma
      b) Respiratory changes: deep, rapid breathing; lungs blow off carbon dioxide to reduce acid load
   3. Treatment and management: Approaches to reduce sodium retention also reduce chloride retention (see this chapter, section II,C,3, for approaches to reducing sodium).
   4. Nursing process
      a) Nursing assessment
         (1) Obtain client history relative to conditions predisposing to hyperchloremia (e.g., head injury, cortisone use).
         (2) Assess for signs and symptoms of hyperchloremia (e.g., weakness, lethargy, deep and rapid breathing).
         (3) Assess for signs of metabolic acidosis.
         (4) Obtain baseline laboratory test values for serum chloride and serum potassium.

III. Potassium (K) imbalances	IV. Calcium (Ca) imbalances	V. Magnesium (Mg) imbalances	VI. Phosphorus (P) imbalances	VII. Chloride (Cl) imbalances

b) Nursing diagnoses: altered health maintenance related to severe dehydration, head injury, excessive use of steroids, or metabolic acidosis

c) Nursing interventions

   (1) Monitor changes in laboratory test values, with emphasis on serum chloride and serum potassium.

   (2) Monitor for worsening signs of hyperchloremia (e.g., increased lethargy).

   (3) Monitor serum carbon dioxide or arterial bicarbonate for metabolic acidosis.

   (4) Keep an accurate record of 24-hour urinary output.

   (5) Instruct the client about a low-sodium diet.

1. A client is admitted to the hospital with syndrome of inappropriate antidiuretic hormone (SIADH). During the initial assessment, which of the following should the nurse expect to find?

   a. Lethargy
   b. Pedal edema
   c. Dilute urine
   d. Fever

2. A 24-year-old schizophrenic is admitted to the hospital with dilutional hyponatremia due to excessive water intake. On admission, the client's serum sodium is 110 mEq/L, and an IV of 250 ml 3% sodium chloride (NaCl) is ordered. During infusion of that IV, the client needs to be monitored closely for:

   a. Fever.
   b. Dyspnea.
   c. Tetany.
   d. Hypotension.

3. Which of the following clients should the nurse identify as being at high risk for hypernatremia?

   a. A construction worker who drinks large amounts of water while working in hot weather
   b. A victim of near drowning in a fresh-water lake
   c. An elderly client with a severe case of Alzheimer's disease
   d. A client with deficient adrenal gland hormone production

4. A client has been using diuretics to lose weight. The client now has a serum potassium level of 2.5 mEq/L. Which of the following nursing diagnoses is most likely to be identified for this client?

   a. Diarrhea related to increased peristalsis
   b. Activity intolerance related to muscle weakness
   c. Altered thought processes related to cerebral edema

d. Hypothermia related to impaired function of the hypothalamus

5. Which of the following items should be removed from the tray of a client being treated for hyperkalemia?

   a. Margarine
   b. White toast
   c. Grapefruit juice
   d. Tea with lemon

6. The nurse taps the facial nerve anterior to the client's left ear and notes twitching of the facial muscles on the left side of the face. This would be documented as a positive:

   a. Chvostek's sign.
   b. Trousseau's sign.
   c. Sulkowitch's test.
   d. Chaddock's sign.

7. A client is admitted with hypercalcemia secondary to thiazide diuretic use. The nursing care plan for this client should include:

   a. Helping the client to eliminate high-sodium foods from the diet.
   b. Teaching the client to avoid juices and vitamins that acidify the urine.
   c. Encouraging the client to ambulate as frequently as tolerable.
   d. Keeping the head of the bed at less than 60° elevation.

8. An 84-year-old woman with a hiatal hernia presents at the emergency room, complaining of nausea and vomiting for the past 2 days. She has been taking Riopan (magaldrate) to control the nausea but without success. Her face is flushed, she reports feeling uncomfortably warm, and her blood pressure is 92/68. Based on her history and symptoms, the nurse should suspect that this client has:

   a. Hypermagnesemia.
   b. Hyperkalemia.
   c. Hyponatremia.
   d. Hypophosphatemia.

9. A client develops severe hypophosphatemia when he misunderstands his prescription and takes too much of his diuretic. He is treated with Neutra-Phos (a phosphorus supplement), 2 capsules BID. The drug will need to be discontinued if he develops:

   a. Respiratory depression.
   b. Severe diarrhea.
   c. Muscle weakness.
   d. Irregular pulse.

10. The client who is diagnosed with hyperphosphatemia is also at high risk for:

    a. Hypernatremia.
    b. Hyperkalemia.
    c. Hypocalcemia.
    d. Hypomagnesemia.

11. A client who has gastroenteritis has been vomiting for 4 days. Upon admission to the hospital, the client's serum chloride is 92 mEq/L, serum sodium is 130 mEq/L, and serum potassium is 3.2 mEq/L. Which of the following orders would be inappropriate for this client?

    a. Chicken bouillon or broth
    b. Gatorade
    c. IV Ringer's solution
    d. Potassium bicarbonate

12. A client is being treated with steroids to control cerebral edema after a head injury. To determine whether the client is developing hyperchloremia, for which change in vital signs should the nurse monitor?

    a. Subnormal temperature
    b. Low blood pressure
    c. Deep, rapid respirations
    d. Slowed pulse rate

ANSWERS

1. **Correct answer is a.** SIADH produces intracellular fluid volume excess, resulting in cerebral edema. Neurologic symptoms, such as lethargy, are prominent.

   b. Because the fluid retained in SIADH is predominantly intracellular, not interstitial, peripheral edema does not occur. Fingerprint edema over the sternum may be seen.
   c. ADH causes the kidneys to conserve, rather than excrete, water. Urine specific gravity is generally greater than 1.012.
   d. Fever is associated with hypernatremia. It is not typical of SIADH.

2. **Correct answer is b.** Dyspnea could be a sign of pulmonary edema—a potential complication of administration of hyperosmolar saline.

   a. Although fever could be a sign of septicemia—a possible complication of any IV therapy—it is not the most likely complication with hyperosmolar saline.
   c. Tetany occurs with hypocalcemia. It is not an adverse effect of hypertonic saline.
   d. As serum sodium increases, osmotic forces produce plasma volume expansion, raising blood pressure. Hypertension, not hypotension, may occur.

3. **Correct answer is c.** The elderly have a decreased response to osmotic stimulation of thirst. Their kidneys are less able to conserve water. Those with impaired cognition are unable to respond appropriately to thirst. Fluid loss without adequate replacement produces hypernatremia.

   a. Both water and sodium are lost in sweat, but this worker is replacing only water and is at risk for hyponatremia.
   b. Saltwater drowning can produce hypernatremia. Freshwater drowning does not.
   d. Both aldosterone and cortisol, which are produced by the adrenal gland, play a role in retention of sodium. Deficiency of these hormones would result in hyponatremia.

4. **Correct answer is b.** Hypokalemia causes muscle weakness: initially in the legs, then the arms, and finally the respiratory muscles.

   a. Paralytic ileus—a clinically significant decrease or general failure of intestinal peristalsis—occurs with hypokalemia. Diarrhea is associated with hyperkalemia.

c. Cerebral edema occurs with hyponatremia. It is not commonly associated with alterations in potassium.

d. Hypothermia is more likely to be associated with fluid volume deficit than with electrolyte imbalances.

5. **Correct answer is c.** Foods and beverages high in potassium should not be served to a client with hyperkalemia. Citrus juices are high in potassium.

a and **b.** Neither of these foods is high in potassium.

d. Tea is not high in potassium. Although lemon juice by the cup would contribute significant potassium to the diet, the amount in a cup of tea would not.

6. **Correct answer is a.** Chvostek's sign is an indicator of tetany, which occurs in hypocalcemia and hypomagnesemia.

b. Trousseau's sign, another indicator of tetany, is the appearance of carpal spasm when a blood pressure cuff on the upper arm is inflated above systolic pressure for 1–5 minutes.

c. Sulkowitch's test is a qualitative test for increased calcium in urine. It is positive in hypercalcemia.

d. Chaddock's sign is flexion of the wrist and fanning of the fingers when the ulnar side of the forearm near the wrist is stroked. It is abnormal in adults and appears on the affected side in hemiplegia. It is not related to electrolyte balance.

7. **Correct answer is c.** Weight bearing and ambulation help to move calcium into bones, reducing the serum calcium level.

a. Sodium promotes calcium excretion, which helps to lower serum calcium level. Unless required by other diagnoses, sodium should not be restricted.

b. A urinary pH lower than 6.5 favors calcium solubility, helping to prevent renal calculi when urinary calcium is increased.

d. Elevation of the head in addition to frequent use of a sitting position helps to prevent urinary stasis, reducing the risk of calculus formation. Sitting should be encouraged.

8. **Correct answer is a.** The elderly often have decreased renal function, which predisposes them to hypermagnesemia. This client is taking Riopan, which contains magnesium. Nausea, vomiting, hypotension, flushed face, and sense of warmth are early signs of magnesium excess.

b. Muscle weakness and paresthesias are the earliest signs of hyperkalemia. Cardiac dysrhythmias may occur.

c. Hyponatremia may cause nausea and vomiting, but the other signs are lethargy, confusion, and muscle twitching.

d. Paresthesias, muscle pain and weakness, and altered mental status are most likely with hypophosphatemia.

9. **Correct answer is b.** Diarrhea is the dose-limiting side effect of phosphate replacement agents.

a and **c.** Respiratory depression and muscle weakness are signs of phosphate depletion. An increased dosage of Neutra-Phos might be indicated.

d. Cardiac dysrhythmias are associated with abnormal serum potassium levels. They are not commonly associated with phosphate replacement therapy.

10. **Correct answer is c.** There is a reciprocal relationship between phosphate and calcium in the body. When serum phosphate levels are elevated, serum calcium levels are lowered.

a, b, and **d.** None of these conditions is clinically related to hyperphosphatemia. Calcium is the only electrolyte whose levels are altered by changes in phosphate level.

11. **Correct answer is d.** Bicarbonate can worsen the chloride deficit. This client may need potassium replacement, but it should

be in the form of potassium chloride to avoid exacerbating the chloride deficit.

a. Bouillon and broth provide both sodium and chloride. Because this client has deficits of both electrolytes, this order would be appropriate.

b. Gatorade is an appropriate electrolyte replacement solution. It provides sodium, potassium, and chloride, all of which are deficient in this client.

c. IV solutions for this client should provide sodium, chloride, and potassium. When hypokalemia and hypochloremia both are present, they need to be corrected simultaneously.

12. **Correct answer is c.** When chloride is increased, bicarbonate is decreased, producing metabolic acidosis. The lungs compensate by increasing carbon dioxide excretion through increased rate and increased depth of respirations.

a. Because sodium and chloride elevations often occur together, fever associated with hypernatremia would more likely occur.

b. Blood pressure elevation would be more likely, because sodium is likely to be elevated when chloride levels are high.

d. Bradycardia is more likely to be associated with hyperkalemia. Chloride alterations are most likely to affect respiratory rate.

4

Acid-Base Imbalances

NURSING HIGHLIGHTS

1. The excess of acid or base ions determines the pH of a solution rather than the absolute hydrogen ion content; carbon dioxide dissolved in serum determines the pH of the blood.

2. Carbon dioxide is regulated by the lungs, the medulla (in the brain), the kidneys, and the buffer systems; each system acts within a different time frame to achieve homeostasis.
3. The fact that systems regulating acid-base balance attempt to compensate for deviations from normal must be considered in interpreting laboratory test results that assess acid-base status.
4. Acid-base imbalances are usually related to an underlying disease state and can appear either as a single imbalance or as multiple imbalances.

GLOSSARY

amphoteric—capable of reacting as an acid or a base
Kussmaul breathing—deep, rapid breathing found in diabetic acidosis

ENHANCED OUTLINE

See text pages
_____

I. Regulation of acid-base balance: Small changes in hydrogen ion concentration cause substantial changes in rates of chemical reactions within the body.

A. Definitions and basic concepts
  1. Hydrogen ion (H^+) concentration of a solution is expressed as pH, the negative logarithm of the amount of H^+ in 1 liter; as H^+ increases, a solution becomes more acidic and pH declines; as H^+ decreases, a solution becomes more alkaline and pH rises.
    a) Measurement of pH
      (1) A liter of neutral solution contains 0.0000001 g of H^+, also written as 10^{-7} or pH 7.
      (2) A neutral solution—neither acid nor base—has the same number of H^+ (acidic) and hydroxyl ions (OH^-, basic); pH 7 is the midpoint on the pH scale.
      (3) An acidic solution has a pH below 7; a basic solution has a pH above 7.
    b) Normal pH of body fluids
      (1) Blood (extracellular fluid [ECF]): adult pH 7.35–7.45, child 7.33–7.43, newborn 7.27–7.47, range compatible with life about 6.8–7.8
      (2) Urine: pH 6.0, but can vary widely
      (3) Gastric juice: pH 1.0–3.5 (very acidic)
      (4) Bile: pH 5.0–6.0

(5) Intracellular fluid: pH 6.9–7.2; not measured clinically; varies in different organs

2. Carbon dioxide (CO_2) acts as an acid in body when dissolved in water (H_2O)

   a) Carbonic acid (H_2CO_3): weak acid formed when CO_2 is dissolved in water of ECF ($H_2O + CO_2 \rightarrow H_2CO_3$); major factor in acid-base balance in the body; as CO_2 concentration increases, H_2CO_3 concentration increases, pH decreases

   b) $PaCO_2$ (partial pressure of CO_2 dissolved in arterial blood): respiratory component of acid-base balance

      (1) Control of $PaCO_2$: Lungs vary amount of CO_2 exhaled or absorbed into blood.

         (a) Deep, rapid respiration: less CO_2 absorbed in blood; blood pH rises

         (b) Shallow, slow respiration: more CO_2 retained by lungs and absorbed into blood; blood pH falls

      (2) Measurement of $PaCO_2$: normal values 35–45 mm Hg adult and child, about 27–40 newborn

   c) Bicarbonate (HCO_3^-): metabolic component of acid-base balance; major base of ECF; accepts protons to form carbonic acid ($HCO_3^- + H^+ \rightarrow H_2CO_3$)

      (1) Types of HCO_3^-: present primarily as sodium bicarbonate ($NaHCO_3$), also as calcium, potassium, and magnesium bicarbonates; HCO_3—sometimes $BHCO_3$—used to represent all bicarbonates

      (2) Measurement of HCO_3: normal values 22–26 mEq/L; some laboratories measure serum CO_2 content rather than HCO_3 (see Nurse Alert, "Understanding CO_2 Laboratory Values")

! NURSE ALERT !

Understanding CO_2 Laboratory Values

Often serum CO_2 content is listed under electrolytes on the laboratory report. This value is a combined measure of all forms of CO_2 in the blood, including CO_2 dissolved in plasma (measured separately as $PaCO_2$), CO_2 as serum bicarbonate (HCO_3), and CO_2 circulating as carbonic acid in the plasma (H_2CO_3). A normal serum CO_2 content measures 22–32 mEq/L. However, because the amount of dissolved CO_2 and H_2CO_3 is small compared with the bicarbonate level, the serum CO_2 content value is, in practice, used to indicate the metabolic component of acid-base balance. Standard bicarbonate (HCO_3) directly measures the metabolic component of acid-base status. $PaCO_2$ measures the respiratory component of acid-base balance. The nurse should understand the differences between those measurements and how they are used in evaluation of acid-base status.

3. Acidity refers to the amount of excess H^+ in solution: in absolute terms, values below pH 7.0; for blood, values below pH 7.35 (lower limit of normal range)
   a) Acid: molecule or ion that can yield a proton to another substance
   b) Acidosis in the body: pH falls below 7.35; depressed central nervous system symptoms leading to disorientation, coma, and death (below pH 6.8); caused by either acid (H^+) excess or alkali (OH^-) deficit
   c) Volatile acid: carbonic acid dissociates readily into CO_2 and H_2O; excreted by the lungs as CO_2 gas to maintain acid-base balance
   d) Nonvolatile acid: a fixed acid (e.g., lactic, pyruvic, or phosphoric acid) in solution that must be excreted in urine; kidneys excrete excess H^+ in form of nonvolatile acid to regulate acid-base balance
4. Alkalinity refers to the amount of excess OH^- in a solution: in absolute terms, pH values over 7.0; for blood, values above 7.45 (upper limit of normal range)
   a) Base (alkali): molecule or ion that can accept a proton from another substance; neutralizes an acid by combining with it to form a neutral salt
   b) Alkalosis in the body: pH rises above 7.45; overstimulation of central nervous system, leading to paresthesia, convulsions, and death (above 7.8); caused by either OH^- excess or H^+ deficit
   c) Base excess (BE): laboratory measurement indicating amount of excess alkali (OH^-) in the blood; normal values range from +2 to –2; reflects metabolic component of acid-base status
5. An acid-base buffer is a compound that can pick up excess H^+ ions, then release them as necessary; prevents large changes in pH when an acid or a base is added to a solution
6. The arterial blood gas (ABG) test measures gases dissolved in arterial blood; it includes $PaCO_2$, HCO_3, and blood pH; used in analysis of acid-base balance

B. Regulatory mechanisms: close regulation of acid-base balance critical; affects most chemical reactions in the body; both rapid and long-term regulation needed to achieve homeostasis
   1. Buffer systems: prevent major changes in pH of body fluids by controlling the availability of hydrogen ions; act within fraction of a second
      a) Bicarbonate-carbonic acid buffer system (carbonate system): most important in the body; maintains acid-base balance 55% of time
         (1) Mechanism of action: Bicarbonate and carbonic acid— present in ECF—trade off H^+ ions to maintain normal blood pH of 7.4 ($HCO_3^- + H^+ \leftrightarrow H_2CO_3$).

      (2) Normal acid-base balance: In ECF, normal HCO_3:H_2CO_3 (bicarbonate:carbonic acid) ratio is 20:1 (i.e., for every 20 OH^- ions there is 1 H^+ ion); ratio determines pH.

      (3) Example—buffering an acid: Hydrochloric acid (HCl; strong acid) is added to a solution containing sodium bicarbonate (buffer); $NaHCO_3$ picks up H^+ from HCl and gives up Na^+ that combines with Cl^- of HCl; this yields H_2CO_3—a weak acid—and sodium chloride ($NaCl$)—a neutral salt ($HCl + NaHCO_3 \rightarrow H_2CO_3 + NaCl$); pH decreases only slightly.

      (4) Example—buffering a base: Sodium hydroxide ($NaOH$; strong base) is added to a solution containing carbonic acid (buffer); H_2CO_3 picks up Na^+ from $NaOH$ and gives up H^+ that combines with OH^- of $NaOH$; this yields $NaHCO_3$—a weak base—and H_2O ($NaOH + H_2CO_3 \rightarrow NaHCO_3 + H_2O$); pH increases only slightly.

  b) Phosphate buffer system: increases amount of sodium bicarbonate ($NaHCO_3$) in ECF; ECF becomes more alkaline; pH increases

      (1) Mechanism of action: In renal tubules, excess H^+ combines with sodium diphosphate (Na_2HPO_4); Na^+ is resorbed, and excess H^+ is excreted in urine.

      (2) Example—phosphate buffering: $Na_2HPO_4 + H^+ \rightarrow Na^+ + NaH_2PO_4$; free Na^+ combines with HCO_3^- to yield $NaHCO_3$, which is resorbed into ECF (pH increases); excess H^+ is excreted in the form of dihydrogen phosphate (NaH_2PO_4).

  c) Hemoglobin-oxyhemoglobin buffer system: maintains same pH value in arterial (oxygenated) and venous (deoxygenated) blood; venous blood higher in CO_2 and HCO_3; acidic oxyhemoglobin in red blood cell (oxygenated blood) takes over some of the anion function of the excess bicarbonate in venous (deoxygenated) blood

  d) Protein buffer system: amphoteric; proteins can exist as acids or bases and bind or release excess H^+ as needed

2. Ion exchange (chloride shift): results from exchange of oxygen and carbon dioxide in red blood cell (RBC); occurs in conjunction with hemoglobin-oxyhemoglobin buffer and respiratory regulation

  a) Mechanism of action: In response to increased serum CO_2 levels, CO_2 enters RBC; bicarbonate ions diffuse out of cell and chloride ions diffuse in to preserve electroneutrality.

  b) Ion exchange: $CO_2 + H_2O \rightarrow H_2CO_3$; $H_2CO_3 \rightarrow HCO_3^- + H^+$; H^+ is buffered by hemoglobin, leaving HCO_3^- free to diffuse out of cell; Cl^- moves into cell to replace negatively charged HCO_3^-

3. Respiratory system: acts within 1–3 minutes

  a) Mechanism of action: Respiratory center in medulla responds to changes in serum CO_2 level and serum pH.

      (1) pH increases: Respiration becomes slow and shallow, causing lungs to retain more CO_2; CO_2 diffuses into blood, creating more carbonic acid (H_2CO_3); pH decreases.

       (2) pH decreases: respiration becomes rapid and deep, causing lungs to force out more CO_2; less H_2CO_3 formed; pH rises

    b) Effectiveness: 50%–75% effective; feedback stimulation to medulla stops when pH approaches normal (about 7.2–7.3)

  4. Renal regulation: responds slowly (many hours or days)

    a) Acidification of phosphate buffer salts (see this chapter, section I,B,1,b, for a discussion of phosphate buffers)

    b) Resorption of bicarbonate: carbonic acid is ionized into hydrogen ions and bicarbonate; HCO_3^- combines with Na^+ in renal tubules and is resorbed into blood, and H^+ is excreted (urine pH decreased); $H_2CO_3 \rightarrow H^+$ (excreted by combining with phosphate salts) $+ HCO_3^-$; $HCO_3^- + Na^+ \rightarrow NaHCO_3$ (resorbed)

    c) Secretion of ammonia (NH_3): almost 50% of excess hydrogen ions excreted this way

       (1) NH_3 unites with hydrochloric acid in renal tubules, forming ammonium chloride, which is excreted ($NH_3 + HCl \rightarrow NH_4Cl$ [excreted]).

       (2) Ammonia can also be converted into urea by the liver and excreted by the kidneys.

  5. Compensation for pH imbalance: regulatory systems attempt to compensate for deviations from normal pH; can result in decrease in signs and symptoms and lead to normal-appearing pH values

C. Identifying acid-base imbalances

  1. Identify imbalance as acidosis or alkalosis: Evaluate pH; less than 7.35 indicates acidosis, and greater than 7.45 indicates alkalosis.

  2. Identify cause of imbalance as respiratory or metabolic.

    a) Acidosis

       (1) If $PaCO_2$ is greater than 45 mm Hg, cause is respiratory.

       (2) If HCO_3 is less than 22 mEq/L, cause is metabolic.

    b) Alkalosis

       (1) If $PaCO_2$ is less than 35 mm Hg, cause is respiratory.

       (2) If HCO_3 is greater than 26 mEq/L, cause is metabolic.

  3. Determine whether imbalance is uncompensated, fully compensated, or partially compensated.

    a) In uncompensated respiratory imbalances, the metabolic component (HCO_3) is normal; in uncompensated metabolic imbalances, the respiratory component ($PaCO_2$) is normal.

    b) In fully compensated imbalances, the pH is normal, but both the respiratory component and the metabolic component are abnormal.

    c) In partially compensated imbalances, all three values are abnormal.

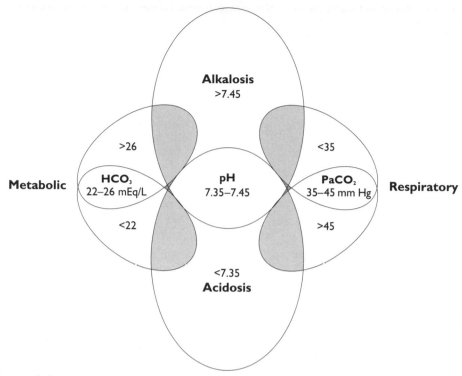

Figure 4–1
Determining Type of Acid-Base Imbalance

II. Metabolic acidosis: an acidotic (low-pH) condition that exists in the body because of production of a deficit of alkali or an excess of nonvolatile (fixed) acids; may be acute or chronic

See text pages
_____

A. Pathophysiology and etiology
1. Serum anion gap (AG): measures difference between the cation sodium and the anions chloride and bicarbonate; gap accounts for unmeasured anions (e.g., anionic proteins, phosphates, sulfates, ketones, lactic acid)
   a) Calculation: $AG = Na^+ - (Cl^- + HCO_3^-)$; normal value 12 ± 2 mEq/L
   b) Interpretation with metabolic acidosis
      (1) High AG: alkali deficit (HCO_3) triggered by increased presence of unmeasured anions (e.g., ketones)
      (2) Normal AG: alkali deficit due to direct loss of HCO_3^- and fluid, inability to form or resorb HCO_3^-, or excess infusion of Cl^- with fluids
      (3) Decreased AG: laboratory error; increased unmeasured cations (e.g., in lithium intoxication); or decreased unmeasured anions (e.g., in hypoalbuminemia)

2. High AG acidosis
   a) Diabetic ketoacidosis: Accumulation of ketones (organic anions formed during abnormal cellular metabolism) causes a decrease in HCO_3^- (to maintain electroneutrality) and an increase in AG.
   b) Starvation (usually in conjunction with alcohol ingestion): Ketones accumulate in blood as in diabetic ketoacidosis.
   c) Lactic acidosis: often due to poor tissue perfusion or hypoxia; increased production or degradation of lactate produces excess lactic acid
      (1) Normal plasma lactate values 0.3–1.3 mEq/L
      (2) Values above 4–5 mEq/L suggest lactic acidosis; levels generally 10–30 mEq/L when lactic acidosis present
      (3) HCO_3^- decreases; AG increases
   d) Uremic acidosis: renal failure; mechanism for conserving Na^+ and H_2O and excreting H^+ fails; HCO_3^- is replaced with sulfate, phosphate, and/or organic acids
   e) Ingestion of toxic substances altering cellular metabolism: salicylates, ethylene glycol, or methyl alcohol
3. Normal AG acidosis
   a) Diarrhea: Direct loss of HCO_3^- and ECF concentrates Cl^-, resulting in hyperchloremic acidosis.
   b) Drainage of pancreatic and biliary fistulas: bicarbonate-rich fluid lost
   c) Urinary diversion into sigmoid colon: increased resorption of chloride by colon at the expense of bicarbonate
   d) Excessive infusion of fluids containing chloride (e.g., 0.9% NaCl); results in hyperchloremic acidosis
   e) Renal tubular acidosis: renal failure marked either by loss of bicarbonate in urine or by inability to produce new bicarbonate

B. Signs and symptoms
   1. Central nervous system changes: depressed central nervous system; headache, apathy, drowsiness, confusion, or coma
   2. Respiratory changes: Kussmaul breathing; lungs compensate by removing more CO_2
   3. Gastrointestinal abnormalities: nausea, vomiting, or abdominal pain
   4. Skin changes: warm and flushed
   5. Summary of laboratory test values associated with metabolic acidosis
      a) pH: <7.35
      b) $PaCO_2$: 35–45 mm Hg (value may fall with compensation)
      c) HCO_3^-: <22 mEq/L
      d) BE: always negative in metabolic acidosis
      e) AG: may be either high or normal
      f) Potassium (K^+): often high (>5 mEq/L)

6. Compensation: may be partial or complete (see this chapter, section I,C,3)
   a) Buffer system acts to neutralize acid and restore pH.
   b) Respiratory system increases amount of CO_2 exhaled through deep, rapid exhalations; $PaCO_2$ decreases.
   c) Renal system acts to excrete more H^+ and retain more HCO_3^-.

C. Treatment and management
   1. Remove cause of acidosis.
   2. Administer parenteral alkali solution (e.g., sodium bicarbonate).
      a) Requires extreme care to avoid hypernatremia, fluid volume overload, and acute hypokalemia
      b) Controversial technique limited to crisis situations in which pH is very low
   3. Restore fluid and electrolyte balance.

D. Nursing process
   1. Nursing assessment
      a) Obtain client history, with emphasis on health problems related to metabolic acidosis (e.g., diabetes, renal disease).
      b) Obtain baseline vital signs, paying special attention to respiration and cardiac functioning.
      c) Assess for signs and symptoms of metabolic acidosis (e.g., weakness, confusion, deep breathing).
      d) Obtain baseline values for ABGs and other laboratory tests, noting abnormalities in serum electrolytes, serum CO_2 content, HCO_3, and blood sugar.
   2. Nursing diagnoses: Most diagnoses involve collaborative diagnosis of underlying causes.
      a) Altered nutrition, less than body requirements, related to starvation, alcoholism, or diabetic ketoacidosis
      b) High risk for injury related to disorientation and confusion
      c) Decreased cardiac output related to severe metabolic acidosis
   3. Nursing interventions
      a) When confusion is present, take safety precautions.
      b) Monitor client's dietary and fluid intake and fluid output.
      c) Monitor laboratory results for changes, especially in ABGs, electrolytes, blood sugar, and serum CO_2 content.
      d) Monitor client for changes in vital signs—especially changes in respiration, cardiac function, and central nervous system.

III. Metabolic alkalosis: an alkalotic condition that exists in the body because of presence of excess alkali or a deficit of nonvolatile acids; may be acute or chronic

See text pages

A. Pathophysiology and etiology
   1. Gastrointestinal abnormalities: vomiting and gastric suction most common cause; loss of HCl in gastric fluid causes increase in HCO_3^-
   2. Hormonal factors: increased adrenocortical hormones (e.g., hyperaldosteronism, Cushing's syndrome)

3. Electrolyte imbalances: hypokalemia; loss of potassium is accompanied by loss of chloride and increase in HCO_3^-
4. Drugs predisposing to metabolic alkalosis: bicarbonate-containing antacids (e.g., Alka-Seltzer); potassium-wasting diuretics (e.g., thiazide, furosemide)

B. Signs and symptoms: may be chronic or acute
   1. Central nervous system changes: paresthesia, dizziness, irritability, or hyperactive reflexes (similar to signs of hypocalcemia)
   2. Respiratory changes: shallow, slow breathing, which conserves CO_2 in lungs
   3. Summary of laboratory test values associated with metabolic alkalosis
      a) pH: >7.45
      b) $PaCO_2$: 35–45 mm Hg (value may rise with compensation)
      c) HCO_3: >26 mEq/L
      d) BE: always positive in metabolic alkalosis
      e) K^+: often low (<3.5 mEq/L)
      f) Urinary chloride: <15 mEq/L when due to vomiting or gastric suction; >20 mEq/L when due to hormonal abnormalities
   4. Compensation
      a) Buffer system responds to neutralize alkali and restore pH.
      b) Respiratory system responds with slow, shallow breathing to conserve CO_2 in lungs; $PaCO_2$ increases.
      c) Renal system excretes more HCO_3^- and retains H^+.

C. Treatment and management
   1. Remove cause of metabolic alkalosis.
   2. Administer parenteral NaCl solution, and restore fluid balance.
   3. Correct potassium deficit with parenteral administration of potassium.

D. Nursing process
   1. Nursing assessment
      a) Obtain client history, with emphasis on health problems related to metabolic alkalosis (e.g., peptic ulcer, vomiting, adrenocortical hormone abnormalities).
      b) Obtain baseline vital signs, paying special attention to respiration.
      c) Assess for signs and symptoms of metabolic alkalosis (e.g., paresthesia, shallow breathing).
      d) Obtain baseline values for ABGs and other laboratory tests, noting abnormalities in serum electrolytes, serum CO_2 content, and HCO_3.

2. Nursing diagnoses: Most diagnoses involve collaborative diagnosis of underlying causes.
   a) Fluid volume deficit related to nasogastric suctioning or vomiting
   b) High risk for injury related to central nervous system excitability
3. Nursing interventions
   a) When hyperexcitability is present, take safety precautions.
   b) Monitor client's fluid intake and fluid output, paying special attention to loss of gastric fluids.
   c) Monitor laboratory results for changes, especially in ABGs, electrolytes, and serum CO_2 content.
   d) Monitor client for changes in vital signs—especially changes in respiration and central nervous system.
   e) Monitor for changes in cardiac rhythm, especially in clients who are taking cardiac glycosides.

IV. Respiratory acidosis: an acidotic condition that exists in the body because of increased carbonic acid in the blood; may be acute or chronic

See text pages _____

A. Pathophysiology and etiology: always due to inadequate ventilation of lungs
   1. Acute respiratory acidosis: blockage of airways due to foreign object; pulmonary edema; overdose of narcotics, anesthetics, or barbiturates; severe pneumonia; cardiac arrest; laryngospasm; or improper mechanical ventilation
   2. Chronic respiratory acidosis: chronic obstructive pulmonary disease (COPD), emphysema, cystic fibrosis, advanced multiple sclerosis, poliomyelitis, or Guillain-Barré syndrome (chest muscles weakened)
   3. Factors predisposing to hypoventilation: obesity, postoperative pain from chest surgery, muscle guarding after abdominal surgery, and abdominal distension from cirrhosis or bowel obstruction

B. Signs and symptoms: more pronounced in acute condition
   1. Central nervous system changes: dizziness, depression, disorientation, muscle twitching, convulsions, or stupor
   2. Respiratory changes: rapid, shallow breathing; difficulty breathing
   3. Cardiac changes: tachycardia and ventricular fibrillation
   4. Skin changes: warm and flushed
   5. Other changes, chronic condition: dull headache or weakness
   6. Summary of laboratory values associated with respiratory acidosis
      a) pH: <7.35
      b) $PaCO_2$: >45 mm Hg
      c) HCO_3: 22–26 mEq/L (value may rise with compensation, which is more probable in chronic conditions)

C. Treatment and management: Aim is to improve ventilation.
   1. Pulmonary hygiene: Suction mucus and drainage fluids from lungs.
   2. Pharmacological agents: bronchodilators (reduce bronchial spasms) and antibiotics (fight infection)

3. Adequate hydration: Keep mucous membranes moist to facilitate removal of secretions.
4. Supplemental oxygen: must be used very carefully in chronic situations, because medulla loses sensitivity to CO_2 levels and relies on oxygen levels to regulate breathing
5. Mechanical ventilation: Use sparingly to allow kidneys to adjust to changes in CO_2 level and avoid alkalosis.

    D. Nursing process
      1. Nursing assessment
        a) Obtain client history, with emphasis on health problems related to respiratory acidosis (e.g., COPD, pneumonia, narcotic use, emphysema).
        b) Obtain baseline vital signs, paying special attention to respiration and cardiac functioning.
        c) Assess for signs and symptoms of respiratory acidosis (e.g., weakness, confusion, tachycardia, difficulty breathing).
        d) Obtain baseline values for laboratory tests, especially noting abnormalities in $PaCO_2$.
      2. Nursing diagnoses
        a) Impaired gas exchange related to inadequate ventilation secondary to pulmonary edema, COPD, or emphysema
        b) Ineffective airway clearance related to thick bronchial secretions, bronchial spasms, or presence of foreign object
        c) Activity intolerance related to difficulty breathing secondary to poor gas exchange
      3. Nursing interventions
        a) When confusion is present, take safety precautions.
        b) Monitor laboratory results for changes, especially in pH and $PaCO_2$.
        c) Monitor client for changes in vital signs—especially changes in respiration (listen for chest sounds), cardiac function, and central nervous system.
        d) Monitor mechanical ventilator when in use.
        e) Monitor oxygen administration when in use.
        f) Elevate head of bed.
        g) Encourage client to perform deep-breathing exercise and to maintain high fluid intake.
        h) Educate client in use of inhaler; assist as needed.
        i) Perform chest clapping to break up mucous when appropriate (e.g., in COPD and cystic fibrosis).

V. Respiratory alkalosis: an alkalotic condition caused by decreased carbonic acid in the blood; may be acute or chronic

See text pages ____

A. Pathophysiology and etiology: always caused by hyperventilation
  1. Psychological causes: extreme anxiety (most common) or hysteria
  2. Disease conditions: brain tumors, meningitis, encephalitis, gram-negative bacteremia, or hyperthyroidism
  3. Other causes: excessive mechanical ventilation, pain, fever, pulmonary emboli, early salicylate poisoning (stimulates respiratory center), pregnancy (increased progesterone level heightens respiratory center's sensitivity to CO_2)

B. Signs and symptoms
  1. Central nervous system changes: dizziness, paresthesia, tetany symptoms, positive Chvostek's and Trousseau's signs, convulsions, or fainting
  2. Respiratory changes: fast, shallow breathing or hyperventilation
  3. Skin changes: sweating and dry mouth
  4. Other changes: palpitations, nausea, vomiting, or blurred vision
  5. Summary of laboratory values associated with respiratory alkalosis
     a) pH: >7.45
     b) $PaCO_2$: <35 mm Hg
     c) HCO_3: 22–26 mEq/L (value may fall with compensation)

C. Treatment and management
  1. Anxiety: Teach patient slow breathing and rebreathing technique; provide prescribed sedation.
  2. Medical conditions: Correct underlying problem.

D. Nursing process
  1. Nursing assessment
     a) Obtain client history, with emphasis on factors relating to respiratory alkalosis (e.g., hysteria, fever, severe infection).
     b) Check for signs and symptoms of respiratory alkalosis (e.g., hyperventilation).
     c) Obtain baseline vital signs.
     d) Obtain ABG values and check for abnormalities.
  2. Nursing diagnoses
     a) Anxiety related to hyperventilation secondary to stress
     b) Ineffective breathing pattern related to hyperventilation and anxiety
  3. Nursing interventions
     a) Encourage patient who is hyperventilating to breathe slowly.
     b) Have client rebreathe expired air by breathing into a paper bag (increases CO_2 content of air being inhaled).
     c) Administer sedative as directed.
     d) Listen to client in emotional distress, and encourage client to seek professional psychological help if indicated.

See text pages

VI. Mixed acid-base imbalances: 2 or more acid-base imbalances occurring simultaneously

A. Metabolic acidosis/respiratory acidosis: cardiopulmonary arrest; lack of oxygen causes production of lactic acid (metabolic acidosis); respiratory arrest causes retention of CO_2 (respiratory acidosis)

B. Metabolic acidosis/respiratory alkalosis: salicylate poisoning; salicylate changes cellular metabolism, resulting in overproduction of organic acids (metabolic acidosis); salicylate stimulation of respiratory center causes hyperventilation (respiratory alkalosis)

C. Metabolic acidosis/metabolic alkalosis: renal failure with vomiting; renal failure causes increased H^+ retention (metabolic acidosis); loss of HCl in gastric fluid causes metabolic alkalosis

D. Metabolic alkalosis/respiratory alkalosis: vomiting during pregnancy; vomiting causes loss of HCl in gastric fluid (metabolic alkalosis); progesterone in pregnancy stimulates medulla, causing hyperventilation (respiratory alkalosis)

E. Metabolic alkalosis/respiratory acidosis: vomiting with chronic obstructive pulmonary disease (causes metabolic alkalosis); COPD causes chronic hypoventilation (respiratory acidosis)

1. To ensure accurate results when a blood specimen is drawn for arterial blood gases (ABGs), the nurse should:

   a. Expel all air from the syringe that will be used to draw the blood.
   b. Refrigerate the specimen until it can be transported to the laboratory.
   c. Discontinue oxygen administration 15 minutes before blood is drawn.
   d. Have the client take 3 or 4 deep breaths before blood is drawn.

2. Which of the following clients is at high risk for metabolic alkalosis?

   a. A client with acute pulmonary edema due to congestive heart failure
   b. A client who has a nasogastric tube to suction following a bowel resection
   c. A client who has a large amount of drainage from a newly created ileostomy
   d. A client with a temperature of 103°F secondary to gram-negative septicemia

3. A client is admitted to the hospital due to methanol poisoning after drinking a home-made alcoholic beverage. The nurse should assess the client for signs of:

   a. Metabolic acidosis.
   b. Metabolic alkalosis.
   c. Respiratory acidosis.
   d. Respiratory alkalosis.

4. For which of the following clients should the nurse anticipate a mixed imbalance involving metabolic acidosis and respiratory alkalosis?

   a. A client who is resuscitated after cardiopulmonary arrest
   b. A client with chronic renal failure who develops vomiting
   c. A client with chronic obstructive pulmonary disease (COPD) who has a nasogastric tube to suction
   d. A client who has taken an overdose of aspirin

5. A client presents with fever and chills. ABG results are pH = 7.51, $PaCO_2$ = 20 mm Hg, HCO_3 = 22 mEq/L, and BE = –2. The nurse recognizes that those results indicate the client has:

   a. Compensated metabolic acidosis.
   b. Compensated respiratory acidosis.
   c. Uncompensated metabolic alkalosis.
   d. Uncompensated respiratory alkalosis.

6. A client has developed metabolic alkalosis due to excessive antacid use. Which of the following nursing diagnoses is most likely to apply to this client?

   a. Ineffective breathing pattern related to respiratory compensation
   b. Constipation related to elevated serum calcium level
   c. Decreased cardiac output related to depressed myocardial contractility
   d. Acute confusion related to impaired neurotransmitter function

7. A client has the following ABG results on admission: pH = 7.2, $PaCO_2$ = 30, HCO_3 = 10, and AG (anion gap) = 38. Possible etiologies for the acid-base imbalance include which of the following?

   a. Excessive respiratory excretion of carbon dioxide
   b. Inability of the kidneys to conserve bicarbonate
   c. Accumulation of lactic acid due to tissue hypoxia
   d. Loss of alkaline intestinal fluids due to diarrhea

8. A client is scheduled for surgical repair of a fractured hip and has a history of COPD. Which complication during surgery should the surgical nurse recognize that this client is at high risk for?

   a. Malignant hyperthermia
   b. Excessive bleeding

c. Ventricular fibrillation

d. Difficulty maintaining anesthetization

9. The nursing care plan for a client with respiratory alkalosis should include:

   a. Elevation of the head of the bed.

   b. Measures to control anxiety.

   c. Encouraging independent ambulation.

   d. A cola drink to control nausea.

10. A client with advanced multiple sclerosis has had a cold for 4 days and has developed respiratory acidosis. The nursing care plan for this client should include:

    a. Providing between-meal snacks that are high in sodium.

    b. Positioning the client only in a supine or side-lying position.

    c. Maintaining bed rest until the cold symptoms are gone.

    d. Encouraging deep breathing and coughing exercises.

11. A client is admitted to the hospital complaining of muscle weakness and paresthesias. Metabolic alkalosis is diagnosed. The nurse should anticipate receiving orders for:

    a. Potassium restriction.

    b. A thiazide diuretic.

    c. IV calcium chloride.

    d. IV normal saline.

12. A client who choked on a piece of meat was resuscitated by a family member using the Heimlich maneuver and then brought to the clinic for evaluation. The client complains of dizziness and a feeling of fullness in the head. The nurse should first:

    a. Encourage the client to take deep breaths.

    b. Have the client sit down and bend over, with the head at knee level.

    c. Start oxygen at 2 liters/minute via face mask.

    d. Notify the physician immediately and bring the crash cart to the room.

ANSWERS

1. **Correct answer is a.** Air in the syringe may alter the partial pressures of gases in the specimen.

   b. The specimen should be placed on ice and delivered to the laboratory immediately.

   c and **d.** Any action that would change the levels of oxygen or carbon dioxide in the client's blood would make the results less useful in evaluating the client's condition.

2. **Correct answer is b.** Loss of gastric fluid is one of the most common causes of metabolic alkalosis.

   a. This client is at high risk for respiratory acidosis.

   c. This client is at high risk for metabolic acidosis.

   d. This client is at high risk for respiratory alkalosis.

3. **Correct answer is a.** Methanol produces metabolites that are acidic anions. This results in a high anion gap (AG) acidosis. The cause is an excess of nonvolatile acids, so the condition is metabolic acidosis.

   b. Metabolic alkalosis is generally related to accumulation of excessive bicarbonate, which does not occur in methanol poisoning.

   c and **d.** This client's acidosis is caused by accumulation of nonvolatile acidic metabolites of methanol; therefore it is metabolic.

4. **Correct answer is d.** Salicylate poisoning leads to overproduction of organic acids, resulting in decreased bicarbonate; this constitutes metabolic acidosis. Salicylates also stimulate the respiratory center, producing hyperventilation, which decreases the carbon dioxide level in the arterial blood; this constitutes respiratory alkalosis.

   a. During cardiopulmonary arrest, hypoxemia produces lactic acidosis, decreasing bicarbonate (metabolic acidosis). However, the pulmonary arrest retains carbon dioxide, producing respiratory acidosis.

b. Acid metabolites are retained in renal failure, causing a decrease in bicarbonate (metabolic acidosis) to maintain electroneutrality. Loss of nonvolatile acids in gastric fluid produces a relative increase in bicarbonate (metabolic alkalosis).

c. Hypoventilation increases the carbon dioxide level in the arterial blood (respiratory acidosis). Loss of nonvolatile acids in gastric fluid produces a relative increase in bicarbonate (metabolic alkalosis).

5. **Correct answer is d.** The pH of 7.51 is alkalotic (normal = 7.35–7.45). Because it is not within the normal range, it is uncompensated. A low $PaCO_2$ is consistent with increased alkalinity of the blood. Therefore it is the cause of the alkalosis.

   a and b. The alkaline pH indicates that this is an alkalosis. Compensatory mechanisms never overcompensate for an acid-base imbalance, so compensation for acidosis cannot produce an alkaline pH.
   c. If this were a metabolic alkalosis, the HCO_3 would be elevated.

6. **Correct answer is a.** To compensate for alkalosis, the lungs reduce their excretion of carbon dioxide through hypoventilation. Hypoventilation can lead to hypoxemia.

   b. Increased protein binding of calcium produces symptoms of hypocalcemia. Constipation occurs in hypercalcemia.
   c. Acidosis depresses myocardial contractility and can cause decreased cardiac output.
   d. Confusion is more likely to occur with acidosis than with alkalosis.

7. **Correct answer is c.** A normal anion gap of 10–14 mEq/L is accounted for by the predominance of chloride and bicarbonate anions in preserving serum electroneutrality. A high AG occurs when large quantities of unmeasured anions, such as lactic acid or ketones, accumulate.

a. Excessive excretion of carbon dioxide would produce alkalosis. In this case, the increased excretion of carbon dioxide is compensatory.
b. If the kidneys are unable to conserve bicarbonate, as in renal tubular acidosis, the chloride level increases and the anion gap is normal.
d. Bicarbonate produces the alkalinity of intestinal fluids. In acidosis due to bicarbonate loss, the chloride level increases and the anion gap is normal.

8. **Correct answer is c.** The client with COPD is at greater risk for respiratory acidosis during anesthesia. Acidosis causes potassium to shift out of cells into the extracellular fluid. Hyperkalemia may cause ventricular fibrillation.

   a. Malignant hyperthermia results from a genetic disorder.
   b. Excessive bleeding would be a risk in clients with deficient clotting factors.
   d. This problem occurs in clients whose tolerance for the drugs that are used to induce anesthesia is increased, usually by chronic alcohol or drug abuse.

9. **Correct answer is b.** Hyperventilation due to anxiety is the most common cause of respiratory alkalosis.

   a. Low carbon dioxide levels in the blood cause cerebral vasoconstriction. Keeping the head flat may improve cerebral blood flow.
   c. Cerebral vasoconstriction causes lightheadedness. The client should have assistance or supervision while ambulating.
   d. Cola-based beverages contain caffeine, which is a respiratory stimulant that could increase hyperventilation.

10. **Correct answer is d.** Deep breathing and coughing mobilize respiratory secretions and promote effective gas exchange, reducing carbon dioxide retention.

    a. Fluid retention due to high sodium levels could cause pulmonary edema and worsen the respiratory acidosis.

b. Semi-Fowler's and high Fowler's positions facilitate lung expansion and improve gas exchange.

c. Because they promote deeper breathing, out-of-bed activities should be encouraged, to blow off retained carbon dioxide.

11. **Correct answer is d.** Dehydration would tend to maintain the alkalosis. Normal saline provides chloride to be absorbed with the sodium, so that excess bicarbonate can be excreted.

a. Hypokalemia due to potassium restriction would help maintain alkalosis.

b. Thiazide diuretics can cause hypokalemia or dehydration, helping to maintain the alkalosis.

c. Symptoms of hypocalcemia are due to increased binding of calcium by serum proteins. Once the alkalosis has been corrected, the calcium will become metabolically active. If calcium is given, the client may develop hypercalcemia as the acid-base balance is restored.

12. **Correct answer is a.** This client has cerebral vasodilation due to sudden elevation of $PaCO_2$. Deep breathing will blow off carbon dioxide, lowering the $PaCO_2$.

b. This position restricts lung expansion. A position with the head elevated helps prevent cerebral edema due to vasodilation.

c. Oxygen will not correct the acidosis or the high $PaCO_2$. Exhaled carbon dioxide can be retained in the mask, allowing the client to rebreathe it and exacerbating the condition.

d. The cause of this client's respiratory acidosis has been corrected, so the symptoms are likely to improve, not worsen.

5

Intravenous Therapy and Tube Feeding

NURSING HIGHLIGHTS

1. Normal renal function is necessary for effective IV therapy.
2. The more hyperosmolar an IV solution, the slower it should be infused and the more frequently the client should be monitored for side effects.
3. The nurse is responsible for administration of IV fluids ordered by the physician, including maintaining both the rate of flow and sterility.
4. Many IV fluids are excellent media for bacterial, fungal, and yeast growth; aseptic practices are essential to prevent contamination.

5. Whenever medications are infused, the frequency of client monitoring must be increased.
6. Tube feedings must be initiated gradually and tapered off slowly to prevent electrolyte imbalances.

GLOSSARY

crystalloid—a substance that, in solution, will readily diffuse through a membrane

refeeding syndrome—a deficit of electrolytes that occurs because of movement of the electrolytes from the extracellular fluid to the intracellular fluid when feeding is resumed after starvation

speed shock—shocklike symptoms that occur when an IV fluid is infused too rapidly, leading to a higher than normal concentration of the substance infused

Trendelenburg position—supine position with head lowered and legs elevated

Valsalva maneuver—client takes a deep breath and bears down, increasing intrathoracic pressure and preventing air from entering the catheter; used in the changing of the tubing at a central venous catheter site

ENHANCED OUTLINE

See text pages
_____

I. Purposes of IV therapy

A. Provision of fluids and electrolytes
1. Maintenance needs: Average adult needs are met by fluid intake of 2000–3000 ml/day, 100 mEq/day of sodium, and 40–60 mEq/day of potassium for short-term maintenance.
2. Previous abnormal fluid losses: Replacement of fluids lost by vomiting, diarrhea, or gastric suctioning prevents fluid volume deficit and restores electrolyte concentrations in body fluids.
3. Continuing abnormal fluid losses: Fluid and electrolyte loss may continue during IV therapy; electrolyte content of IV fluids can be adjusted to replenish losses.

B. Provision of nutrition: Supplemental IV nutrition meets some nutritional needs; total parenteral nutrition (TPN) meets all nutritional needs.

C. Provision of blood and blood components: Whole blood, packed red blood cells (RBCs), plasma, platelets, white blood cells, albumin, and various blood factors can be administered IV.

D. Administration of medication: IV therapy is the preferred vehicle for effective administration of many medications.

Solution mEq/L:	Na⁺	K⁺	Ca⁺⁺	Cl⁻	Lactate
Hypo-osmolar					
0.2% NaCl	34	0	0	34	0
Half-strength saline (0.45% NaCl)	77	0	0	77	0
Iso-osmolar					
Normal saline (0.9% NaCl)	154	0	0	154	0
Lactated Ringer's	130	4	3	109	28
M/6 sodium lactate	167	0	0	0	167
Dextrose 2.5% in half-strength saline	77	0	0	77	0
Dextrose 5% in water	0	0	0	0	0
Hyperosmolar					
Hyperosmolar saline (3% NaCl)	513	0	0	513	0
(5% NaCl)	856	0	0	856	0
Dextrose 5% in half-strength saline	77	0	0	77	0
Dextrose 5% in normal saline	154	0	0	154	0
Dextrose 5% in lactated Ringer's	130	4	3	109	28

Figure 5–1
Electrolyte Content of Common IV Solutions

II. IV solutions

A. Source of free water and kcal
1. 5% hydrated dextrose (D_5W) is iso-osmolar, but dextrose is rapidly metabolized, resulting in release of free water (see Nurse Alert, "Intravenous Use of D_5W").
2. 1 liter of D_5W provides 170 kcal (3.4 kcal/g of dextrose) and helps prevent cellular catabolism caused by starvation.
3. Hydrated dextrose is also available in 2.5%, 10% ($D_{10}W$), 20%, and 50% concentrations (higher concentrations used in TPN).

See text pages
_____

! NURSE *ALERT* !

Intravenous Use of D_5W

Distilled water—a hypo-osmolar solution—cannot be given intravenously to provide free water, because its infusion results in hemolysis of RBCs. 5% dextrose in water (D_5W)—an iso-osmolar solution—is commonly given as a source of free water. The dextrose is rapidly metabolized to carbon dioxide and water without RBC hemolysis. However, D_5W is never used alone to expand extracellular fluid volume, because much of the free water moves out of the intravascular space and into cells. With continuous administration of D_5W, serum osmolality decreases. Alternate use of D_5W and dextrose in normal saline can prevent that problem.

B. Crystalloids (electrolytes): Iso-osmolar solutions contain about 300 mEq/L of electrolytes, hypo-osmolar solutions less than 240 mEq/L, and hyperosmolar solutions greater than 340 mEq/L.
  1. Iso-osmolar, isotonic, or normal saline: 0.9% sodium chloride (NaCl); contains 154 mEq/L each of sodium and chloride; provides excess sodium and chloride, but no other electrolytes and no kcal; may have 5% or 10% dextrose added for kcal (makes solution hyperosmolar)
  2. Hypo-osmolar saline: 0.2% NaCl and 0.45% NaCl (half-strength saline) provide lower level of electrolytes with free water needed for kidneys to eliminate solutes; may have dextrose (2.5% or 5%) added for kcal (makes 0.2% NaCl iso-osmolar; makes 0.45% NaCl iso-osmolar or hyperosmolar, respectively)
  3. Hyperosmolar saline: 3% and 5% NaCl are dangerously hyperosmolar; used sparingly only to treat severe hyponatremia
  4. Lactated Ringer's: roughly iso-osmolar; contains multiple electrolytes in same concentration as plasma; lacks magnesium, phosphate, and adequate potassium; used for maintenance and to treat hypovolemia, burns, fluid lost as diarrhea, and mild metabolic acidosis; may have 5% dextrose added for kcal (makes solution hyperosmolar)
  5. Ringer's solution: iso-osmolar; lacks lactate; used for clients unable to metabolize lactic acid; may have 5% dextrose added for kcal (hyperosmolar)
  6. M/6 sodium lactate: iso-osmolar; supplies sodium without chloride; used for treatment of metabolic acidosis in clients without liver disease
  7. 2.14% ammonium chloride: used cautiously to correct metabolic alkalosis in clients without liver or kidney disease
  8. Multiple electrolyte solutions: iso-osmolar or hypo-osmolar (hypo-osmolar solutions provide free water); commercially available under many different brand names (e.g., Plasma-Lyte 56, Plasma-Lyte 148); variations available to address specific electrolyte and fluid imbalances

C. Colloids (plasma expanders): fluids containing protein or starch molecules that remain uniformly distributed and do not form a true solution; increase fluid volume by increasing plasma oncotic pressure and drawing fluid into intravascular space; can stay in vascular system for several days
  1. Albumin: prepared from human donor plasma; used for restoration or maintenance of blood volume after acute blood loss, nonhemorrhagic shock, burns after 24 hours when hypoproteinemia is present, hepatic failure, or protein-losing nephropathy; 5% albumin osmotically equivalent to plasma; 25% albumin also used; may cause allergic reaction or fluid volume overload

2. Dextran: polysaccharide that behaves like a colloid; interferes with blood clotting, typing, and cross matching (see Nurse Alert, "Dextran and Blood Cross Matching"); improves microcirculation by reducing blood aggregation in capillaries; Dextran 40 stays in vascular system 4–6 hours, Dextran 70 about 20 hours; should not be used in clients with severe dehydration (because it draws more water out of cells), renal disease, thrombocytopenia, or active hemorrhage; may cause allergic reaction

3. Hetastarch: synthetic starch colloid and plasma expander; increases blood-clotting time; small chance of allergic reaction; cannot be used in clients with renal or heart disease or fluid retention; may cause fluid volume overload

D. Blood and blood components: whole blood, packed RBCs, plasma, platelets, white blood cells, albumin, and blood factors II, VII, VIII, IX, and X (see this chapter, section IV, for a discussion of blood transfusion)

E. Hyperosmolar solutions: used for TPN (see this chapter, section V)

F. Incompatible admixtures: Some medications and parenteral solutions cannot be mixed; if in doubt, seek advice from hospital pharmacist.
  1. Physical incompatibilities: produce a change in color, haze, precipitate, or effervescence (e.g., sodium bicarbonate and calcium salts produce calcium carbonate precipitate); discard IV mixture
  2. Chemical incompatibilities: no visible change, but often involve incompatibility of pH; medication can be degraded (e.g., when epinephrine is administered with sodium bicarbonate, epinephrine is neutralized)

III. IV procedures: Physician prescribes amount, type, rate, and route of administration; nurse is responsible for establishing and maintaining correct administration and maintaining sterility.

See text pages
_____

A. IV equipment
  1. Infusion systems
    a) Plastic bottle or bag: popular in United States
      (1) Advantages: lighter, easier to store; breakage not a concern; no air enters system, thereby reducing contamination and air

emboli; no rubber bushing, thereby reducing particulate matter

    (2) Disadvantages: accidental puncture possible

  b) Glass bottle closed system: partial vacuum, air vents required, only filtered air enters

  c) Glass bottle open system: partial vacuum, unfiltered air enters through plastic tube

2. Administration sets: Correct use of sets varies by type and manufacturer; read directions, and have set demonstrated.

  a) Macro (regular) IV administration sets: basic set; output ranges from 8 to 20 drops(gtt)/ml(cc) with various manufacturers

  b) Microdrip (pediatric) IV administration sets: maintains flow at minimal rate; output ranges from 50 to 60 drops/ml

  c) Check-valve IV administration sets: Check valve allows secondary or piggybacked IV fluid to be delivered without mixing with primary fluid; primary bottle must be hung lower than secondary bottle.

  d) Nonpolyvinyl chloride IV administration sets: circumvents the absorption of fat emulsions and of some drugs into tubing walls (problem with polyvinyl chloride tubing)

3. Filters: prevent passage of particulate matter (e.g., glass, precipitates, rubber, fungi, bacteria) into vein; available in sizes from 5.0 to 0.22 μ; 0.22-μ size eliminates bacteria and air; use varies

4. Electronic infusion devices

  a) Controller: electronic device that regulates flow rate; gravity delivers solution

  b) Infusion pump: uses positive pressure to deliver accurate volume; three types—syringe pump, volumetric pump, and nonvolumetric pump

5. Cannulas: used for introduction of IV fluids into veins

  a) Metal cannula: traditional stainless steel needle; rarely used today

  b) Winged-tip (butterfly or scalp-vein) needle: consists of a metal cannula (gauges 16–26), flexible plastic wings, and plastic hub; needle and tubing are bonded into single unit; easy to secure; difficult to rotate; used for children and the elderly

6. Catheters

  a) Over-the-needle catheter (ONC): bevel of needle extends beyond catheter; catheter guided off needle into vein; gauges 8–22; good for rapid infusions; more comfortable for client; many types commercially available

  b) Through-the-needle catheter: opposite of ONC; catheter rests in needle and is guided through needle into vein; gauges 8–22; long and narrow; best for prolonged infusions

c) In-lying catheter: introduced by cut down of vein (minor surgery performed by physician)

d) Central-venous catheter: used in long-term IV therapy to measure central-venous pressure, in TPN to infuse multiple fluids (1–4 lumens running full length of catheter), and in IV administration of medications to infuse irritating medications (e.g., chemotherapeutic medications); radiopaque; inserted into subclavian, internal jugular, femoral, or antecubital vein in operating room (Hickman, Broviac, and Groshong catheters); complications include pneumothorax, air embolism, phlebitis, infection, cardiac dysrhythmia, and impaired circulation

e) Fully implanted catheter: used in long-term IV therapy; no dangling tubes; implanted under skin in operating room; less chance of infection; better for client lifestyle

B. Peripheral IV therapy

1. Site selection: Factors include suitable location, condition of veins, purpose of infusion, duration of therapy, and restrictions based on client's clinical status.
   a) Choose best vein in nondominant arm.
   b) Avoid leg veins (increased chance of thrombosis or phlebitis).
   c) Avoid arms affected by stroke or mastectomy.

2. Cannula or catheter selection: Factors include purpose of infusion; duration of therapy; condition, size, and availability of veins; and client's age and clinical status.

3. Insertion: Always use universal precautions.
   a) Distension of veins: Avoid tight tourniquet or exercising muscle when drawing sample for serum electrolytes.
   b) Skin preparation: Scrub with 70% alcohol or povidone-iodine.
   c) Insertion: Procedure varies with type of cannula; normally, bevel of needle points up; skin is pierced ½ inch below and to the side of spot where needle enters vein; check surrounding area for displaced fluid flow from incorrect insertion; discontinue in presence of swelling; anchor set securely.
   d) Site maintenance: Apply antimicrobial and sterile dressing after insertion; observe frequently for signs of infection, infiltration, cannula occlusion, or phlebitis.
   e) Rotation: Change IV site every 2–3 days; needles left in longer than 72 hours greatly increase risk of phlebitis.

C. Flow rates

1. General principles
   a) Regulation of flow is important in preventing overhydration (see this chapter, section III,D,2,f).
   b) Hyperosmolar fluids are infused more slowly than iso-osmolar fluids.
   c) Flow rate varies with type of administration set used, with manufacturer, and with type of fluid infused.
   d) If IV flow stops, catheter should be removed; forcible irrigation can dislodge fatal blood clots.

2. Calculation of flow rate: Nurse needs to know how many drops per minute to administer.
   a) Total volume: determined by physician's order
   b) Total time in minutes: To convert into minutes the hours given in physician's order, multiply by 60.
   c) Drops(gtt)/ml(cc): provided by administration set manufacturer
   d) Flow rate $= \dfrac{\text{total volume in ml} \times \text{drops/ml}}{\text{time in hours} \times 60 \text{ minutes/hour}}$
   e) Example: 2500 ml to be run for 24 hours with an administration set infusing 15 drops/ml:

   $$\frac{2500 \text{ ml} \times 15 \text{ drops/ml}}{24 \text{ hours} \times 60 \text{ minutes/hour}} = \frac{37,500}{1440} = 26 \text{ drops/min}$$

3. Factors influencing gravity flow: change in cannula position, height of infused solution container above client (the greater the distance between client and container, the faster the flow), patency of cannula (blood clots can slow flow), venous spasm (slows flow), plugged air vent (stops flow), clogged filter, crying in infants (raises venous pressure and slows flow), and presence of phlebitis or undetected infiltration (slows flow)

D. Complications: Clients receiving IV therapy need frequent monitoring.
   1. Local
      a) Infiltration: collection of IV fluid in subcutaneous tissue
         (1) Cause: improper vein puncture; dislodgment of needle (common)
         (2) Signs: edema at injection site, pain at site, or decreased rate of flow
         (3) Detection: place two fingers on vein 3–4 inches above injection site, and press; if flow stops, no infiltration; if flow unchanged, infiltration
         (4) Intervention: Remove cannula; educate client concerning care of affected extremity; restrain hyperactive client; secure device appropriately.
      b) Hematoma: blood enters tissues through puncture in vein wall; apply adequate pressure after device is removed until all bleeding stopped
      c) Phlebitis: inflammation of vein
         (1) Cause: chemical, due to irritant properties of IV solution (e.g., low pH); mechanical when cannula moves too much inside vein; infection when cannula left in too long (more than 72 hours)
         (2) Signs: heat, redness, swelling, and pain near venipuncture site; with thrombophlebitis (blood clot and inflammation), hardness and tenderness of veins and decreased infusion flow

        (3) Prevention: Maintain sterile conditions; change solution container and administration sets at recommended intervals; rotate venipuncture sites; anchor cannula securely.

2. Systemic
  a) Pyrogenic reaction: rapid-onset fever
    (1) Cause: introduction of foreign proteins into the body
    (2) Signs: abrupt rise in temperature with chills (usually about 30 minutes after infusion begins), backache, headache, nausea, vomiting, vascular collapse, hypotension, and cyanosis
    (3) Interventions: Stop infusion; check vital signs; notify physician.
  b) Systemic infection (sepsis): similar to pyrogenic reaction, although onset slower; prevent by rigorous use of aseptic technique
  c) Speed shock
    (1) Cause: infusion of drugs given too rapidly; a high concentration accumulates in the body
    (2) Signs: shocklike symptoms; decreased blood pressure, fainting, and tachycardia
    (3) Prevention: Infuse medications slowly; stop immediately if shocklike symptoms occur.
  d) Air embolism: serious complication
    (1) Cause: air entering circulatory system; more likely to be associated with central-vein cannulization than peripheral-vein cannulization
    (2) Signs: pallor, fainting, tachycardia, decreased blood pressure, cough, and difficulty breathing
    (3) Prevention: Examine for defects all infusion bottles and bags as well as all administration sets; secure all connections tightly; stop infusion before bottle and tubing are empty; have client, in Trendelenburg position, perform Valsalva maneuver during tubing changes of central line.
    (4) Intervention: Place client on left side in modified Trendelenburg position to trap embolism in right atrium and prevent its entry into lung; notify physician.
  e) Pulmonary embolism: serious complication
    (1) Cause: thrombus (blood clot) breaks loose in peripheral vein and moves into pulmonary artery; inappropriate irrigation of blocked cannula or inappropriate venipuncture technique
    (2) Signs: restlessness, chest pain, cough, difficulty breathing, and tachycardia
    (3) Prevention: Never forcibly irrigate cannula to reestablish flow; avoid veins in lower extremities for IV therapy.
    (4) Intervention: Administer oxygen, analgesics, anticoagulants, and IV fluids on physician's order.
  f) Circulatory overload (i.e., fluid volume excess, overhydration): pulmonary edema and/or congestive heart failure; signs include shortness of breath, increased respiratory rate, coughing, cyanosis, chest rales, and neck vein engorgement

      g) Allergic and untoward reactions
        (1) Causes: allergic reaction to infused blood products or medications; certain medications irritate veins (e.g., potassium, antineoplastic drugs, low-pH drugs)
        (2) Interventions: Check compatibility charts before adding medication to IV solutions (see this chapter, section II,F, for more on incompatible admixtures); mix medications and IV solutions thoroughly; remain with client 10–15 minutes to observe reactions.

See text pages

IV. Blood transfusion

A. Indications for blood transfusion: altered oxygen-carrying capacity of blood, depleted blood components, and depleted extracellular fluid volume

B. Metabolic complications of blood transfusion
  1. Immune-mediated reaction: Blood must be typed and cross matched.
  2. Transfused infections: AIDS, malaria, and hepatitis
  3. Fluid and electrolyte imbalances
    a) Hyperkalemia: potassium level increases in stored whole blood as RBCs break down; storage life of refrigerated whole blood 35 days, frozen RBCs and plasma 3 years, and separated platelets 3 days; old blood inappropriate for clients already at risk for hyperkalemia
    b) Hypocalcemia: Excess citrate from blood preservative (citrate-phosphate-dextrose) may combine with ionized calcium in client's blood; most at risk are infants, adults with liver disease, clients with osteoporosis, and clients transfused too rapidly.

See text pages

V. Total parenteral nutrition (TPN): Enteral feedings are preferred over TPN, or hyperalimentation.

A. Indications for TPN: enteral feedings inadequate to supply nutritional needs; enteral feedings not tolerated; generally, indications anticipated for more than 7–10 days
  1. Negative nitrogen balance: severe malnutrition, extensive surgical trauma, or body in anabolic state (e.g., AIDS, metastatic cancer)
  2. Gastrointestinal tract abnormalities: difficulty chewing and swallowing (dysphagia), malabsorption syndrome, fistulas, major bowel resection, ulcerative colitis, and Crohn's disease
  3. Hypermetabolic states: sepsis and burns

B. Composition of TPN: Parenteral solution must meet all of a client's nutritional needs in a balanced way.

1. Proteins (as amino acids): 4 kcal/g; necessary to restore positive protein balance and build new cells (anabolism)
2. Hydrated dextrose (glucose): 3.4 kcal/g; main source of kcal; must provide adequate kcal from dextrose, or proteins will be metabolized for energy; necessary for normal fat metabolism; because solutions higher than 10% dextrose cannot be infused peripherally (phlebitis), central-venous catheter must be used
3. Fat: 9 kcal/g; necessary to maintain cell membrane integrity and carry fat-soluble vitamins (A, D, E, K); best tolerated are 10% or 20% soybean or safflower oil emulsions
4. Vitamins: water-soluble vitamins not stored by body; require daily replacement
5. Minerals: Requirements vary with underlying disease; clients receiving long-term TPN (more than 30 days) require trace-element supplements (e.g., zinc, copper, chromium, iodine, manganese).

C. Delivery of TPN
   1. Central-venous delivery: preferable because large volume of blood dilutes hyperosmolar TPN solution; essential in clients receiving long-term TPN; infusion must be increased gradually (see this chapter, section III,A,6,d, for a discussion of central-venous catheters)
   2. Peripheral delivery: limited to clients who are expected to reestablish enteral nutrition in 3–7 days; final dextrose concentration cannot exceed 10% (higher irritates veins); fat emulsions required to supply sufficient caloric intake

D. Metabolic complications of TPN
   1. Abnormal glucose levels
      a) Hyperglycemia: occurs if initial flow rate too high
         (1) Pathophysiology and etiology: excess dextrose infusion, inadequate insulin, glucocorticoid administration, or sepsis
         (2) Signs and symptoms: thirst; polyuria; hot, flushed skin; fatigue; glycosuria; and elevated blood glucose
         (3) Treatment and management: slow flow rate; administer exogenous insulin, as ordered
      b) Hypoglycemia: occurs if nutrition support ends abruptly
         (1) Pathophysiology and etiology: abrupt end of high-concentration dextrose solution; excessive insulin
         (2) Signs and symptoms: weakness, hunger, nervousness, irritability, headaches, blurred vision, and sweating
         (3) Treatment and management: Administer 10% dextrose solution.
      c) Hyperglycemic hyperosmolar nonketotic (HHNK) coma (see Chapter 12 for detailed coverage)
   2. Fluid and electrolyte imbalances: often due to underlying disease, but may be initiated (e.g., refeeding syndrome) or aggravated by TPN
      a) Potassium imbalances (see Chapter 3, section III,B and C, for a discussion of signs, symptoms, and treatment)

      (1) Hypokalemia: related to potassium shift from extracellular fluid (ECF) to intracellular fluid (ICF); enhanced by administration of insulin; close monitoring of serum potassium levels required at start of TPN

      (2) Hyperkalemia: addition of excess potassium to TPN solution; excess intake from other sources; clients with impaired renal function at highest risk

  b) Phosphorus imbalances (see Chapter 3, section VI,B and C, for a discussion of signs, symptoms, and treatment)

      (1) Hypophosphatemia: common imbalance, especially in clients receiving hypertonic dextrose with insulin; increased phosphate uptake by cells produces serum phosphate deficit

      (2) Hyperphosphatemia: not common; addition of excess phosphates to TPN solution; clients with impaired renal function at highest risk

  c) Magnesium imbalances (see Chapter 3, section V,B and C, for a discussion of signs, symptoms, and treatment)

      (1) Hypomagnesemia: caused by shift of magnesium from ECF to ICF, inadequate replacement via TPN solution, or excessive calcium (causes magnesium to be excreted)

      (2) Hypermagnesemia: addition of excess magnesium to TPN solution; clients with impaired renal function at highest risk

  d) Calcium imbalances (see Chapter 3, section IV,B and C, for a discussion of signs, symptoms, and treatment)

      (1) Hypocalcemia: due to malnutrition, decreased serum albumin, or hypomagnesemia

      (2) Hypercalcemia: due to metabolic imbalance—associated with long-term TPN—that releases ionized calcium from bone or vitamin D supplements in excess of need

3. Acid-base imbalances: usually result from effects of underlying disease on metabolism of TPN solution components

  a) Metabolic acidosis (see Chapter 4, section II): results from excess hydrogen ions released from complete metabolism of amino acids containing sulfur (e.g., methionine, cysteine, cystine)

  b) Metabolic alkalosis (see Chapter 4, section III): results from conversion of excess acetate in TPN solution to bicarbonate

  c) Respiratory acidosis (see Chapter 4, section IV): caused by increased carbon dioxide production due to excessive carbohydrate infusion; clients with impaired pulmonary function at greatest risk

4. Trace-element disturbances: in clients receiving long-term TPN

  a) Zinc deficiency

      (1) Pathophysiology and etiology: increased loss of zinc in catabolic illnesses; increased demand during tissue building

    (2) Signs and symptoms: diarrhea, delayed wound healing, mental changes, abnormalities in taste and smell, and dermatitis

    (3) Treatment and management: Add zinc to parenteral solution; excess can cause zinc toxicity, especially in clients with renal failure.

  b) Copper deficiency: Hypochromic anemia or neutropenia usually occurs after months of TPN; serum copper level may drop below normal within weeks.

  c) Chromium deficiency: causes glucose intolerance, mental confusion, or peripheral sensory neuropathy; reversible with addition of chromium to parenteral solution

  d) Selenium and molybdenum deficiencies: clinical manifestations uncommon, resolve with supplementation

5. Other complications: All of the complications described in section III,D of this chapter can occur during administration of TPN.

E. Nursing process: same for central-venous or peripheral-venous delivery of TPN

  1. Nursing assessment

     a) Assess vital signs and obtain baseline values.

     b) Evaluate medical records for conditions predisposing to fluid or clcctrolyte imbalances.

     c) Obtain baseline values for laboratory tests, including electrolytes, blood urea nitrogen (BUN), creatinine, and serum glucose.

     d) Confirm x-ray report that central-venous catheter is properly located.

     e) Understand physician's orders relative to type of solution, volume, and time of infusion.

     f) Evaluate factors related to selection of administration set, cannula, and administration site (e.g., age of client, condition of veins, rate and volume to be infused, type of solution to be infused).

  2. Nursing diagnoses

     a) High risk of infection related to TPN therapy requiring dressing and tubing changes

     b) High risk of fluid volume overload related to inappropriate rate of IV administration or underlying disease

     c) Altered comfort related to therapy using central-venous catheter

     d) Impaired gas exchange related to introduction of air embolism when inserting, removing, or changing central-venous lines or changing TPN solutions

  3. Nursing interventions

     a) Check type, volume, osmolality, and integrity of IV solutions ordered by physician.

     b) Check for incompatible admixtures; seek assistance from hospital pharmacist if necessary.

     c) Monitor vital signs, being especially alert to changes in pulmonary and cardiac functions.

d) Monitor laboratory test results, noting changes.
e) Monitor blood glucose level frequently.
f) Maintain sterility of IV solution and equipment.
g) Monitor and maintain IV lines; flow rate must be maintained; follow institutional policy on monitoring.
h) Change IV tubing and central-venous dressings every 24–48 hours in accordance with institutional policy.
i) Observe client for signs of infection.
j) Monitor client's fluid intake and output.
k) Monitor client's nutritional status and daily weight.
l) Monitor client's complaints of pain and discomfort (often indicative of clot formation or pulmonary embolism).
m) Respond to specific complications as indicated in section III,D of this chapter.

VI. Tube feeding: enteral feeding

See text pages

A. Indications for tube feeding: dysphagia; provides nutrition for clients with functional gastrointestinal tracts who cannot consume adequate kcal

B. Composition of enteral formulas
   1. Nutrients: proteins, carbohydrates, fats, minerals, vitamins, and electrolytes; can be varied to meet specific needs (e.g., burns, trauma); many commercial brands available (e.g., Ensure, Entralife, Resource, Vitaneed)
   2. Osmolality: determined primarily by concentration of proteins, carbohydrates, and electrolytes; information on osmolality provided by manufacturer
      a) Osmolality determines renal solute load; increased solute load requires increased free water for excretion.
      b) Commercial products range from iso-osmolar (e.g., Isolan, 300 mOsm/kg) to highly hyperosmolar (e.g., Magnacal, 590 mOsm/kg).
      c) Hyperosmolar formulas are diluted to iso-osmolar strengths at beginning of tube feedings and then gradually increased.
      d) Hyperosmolar formulas can slow gastric emptying, leading to nausea, vomiting, and diarrhea.
   3. Electrolytes: Commercial formulas have standard concentrations that often fail to meet the electrolyte needs related to client's underlying disease.
   4. Variant formulations: commercial formulas available for clients with specific problems such as trauma, burns, renal failure, hepatic failure, or respiratory failure; altered nutritional content

Product (manufacturer)	mOsm/kg	% Kcal from Carbohydrate	% Kcal from Protein	% Kcal from Fat	Use Indication
Ensure (Ross)	470	55	14	32	Tube/oral feeding
Magnacal (Sherwood)	590	50	14	36	Tube/oral feeding
Resource (Sandoz)	430	54	14	32	Tube/oral feeding
Entralife (Corpak)	300	55	14	31	Tube feeding
Isolan (Elan Pharma)	300	54	15	31	Tube feeding
Vitaneed (Sherwood)	300	48	16	36	Tube feeding
Impact (Sandoz)	375	53	22	25	Metabolic stress
Traumacal (Mead Johnson)	490	38	22	40	Metabolic stress
Accupep HPF (Sherwood)	490	76	16	9	Gastrointestinal dysfunction
Peptamen (Clintec)	270	51	16	33	Gastrointestinal dysfunction
Amin-Aid (Kendall McGaw)	700	75	4	21	Renal dysfunction
Nepro (Ross)	635	43	14	43	Renal dysfunction
Hepatic–Aid II (Kendall McGaw)	560	57	15	28	Hepatic dysfunction
Travasorb Hepatic (Clintec)	600	77	11	12	Hepatic dysfunction
Nutrivent (Clintec)	450	27	18	55	Pulmonary dysfunction
Pulmocare (Ross)	520	28	17	55	Pulmonary dysfunction

Figure 5–2
Enteral Formulas

C. Metabolic complications of tube feeding
   1. Abnormal glucose levels (same as section V,D,1 of this chapter)
   2. Fluid and electrolyte imbalances
      a) Sodium imbalance (see Chapter 3, section II,B and C, for a discussion of signs, symptoms, and treatment)
         (1) Hypernatremia: results when clients receive hyperosmolar feedings with inadequate free water; elderly and children most at risk (difficulty concentrating urine)
         (2) Hyponatremia: associated with excessive enteral intake of water (e.g., formula diluted unnecessarily, excessive tube flushing), excessive D_5W infusion (releases free water), and

excess water retention (e.g., syndrome of inappropriate antidiuretic hormone [SIADH])

b) Potassium imbalances (see Chapter 3, section III,B and C, for a discussion of signs, symptoms, and treatment)

(1) Hypokalemia: caused by movement of potassium from ECF to ICF; enhanced by insulin administration, diarrhea, and use of potassium-wasting diuretics; common—found in up to 50% of clients

(2) Hyperkalemia: caused by excess administration of potassium; enhanced risk in clients with metabolic acidosis or renal failure

c) Phosphorus imbalances (see Chapter 3, section VI,B and C, for a discussion of signs, symptoms, and treatment)

(1) Hypophosphatemia: caused by phosphate shift into cells for use in glucose and protein metabolism

(2) Hyperphosphatemia: occurs primarily in clients with renal failure or other underlying disease or both

d) Hypomagnesemia: caused by increased demand during cellular anabolism or inadequate replacement therapy (see Chapter 3, section V,B, for a discussion of signs, symptoms, and treatment)

e) Fluid-volume overload: related to excess sodium retention or inadequate water excretion

f) Fluid volume deficit: associated with hyperglycemia when clients with insulin resistance receive high-carbohydrate formula (see Chapter 12 for a discussion of HHNK coma)

3. Zinc deficiency: Clients develop skin rashes that disappear with addition of zinc to formula.

4. Diarrhea: common complication related to osmolality of formula, volume, rate, and site of delivery (e.g., gastric or intestinal), medications, and general health of client; incidence increases as health status declines; increases risk of electrolyte imbalances

D. Nursing process

1. Nursing assessment

a) Assess vital signs, and obtain baseline values.

b) Evaluate medical records for conditions predisposing to fluid or electrolyte imbalances; assess hydration status of client.

c) Obtain baseline values for laboratory tests, including electrolytes, BUN, creatinine, and serum glucose.

d) Understand physician's orders relative to type of formula, formula osmolality, volume, and rate of delivery.

e) Evaluate factors related to selection of formula and site of delivery (e.g., health status of client, underlying disease, factors predisposing to fluid and electrolyte imbalances).

2. Nursing diagnoses
   a) Fluid volume deficit with hypernatremia related to hyperosmolar tube feedings or inadequate water supplements or both
   b) Fluid volume excess secondary to renal failure, SIADH, or congestive heart failure
   c) Alteration in bowel elimination, diarrhea, related to rapid administration of hyperosmolar formula, contamination of formula
   d) Alteration in electrolyte balance of potassium, phosphorus, and/or magnesium; concentration below normal limits; related to refeeding syndrome or diarrhea
3. Nursing interventions
   a) Check type, volume, osmolality, and integrity of feeding formula.
   b) Monitor vital signs, being especially alert to changes in pulmonary and cardiac functions as indications of fluid-volume changes.
   c) Monitor laboratory test results, noting changes especially in BUN:creatinine ratio (an indicator of fluid volume deficit).
   d) Monitor blood glucose level frequently, especially once treatment has been initiated.
   e) Monitor fluid intake, output, and urine concentration.
   f) Monitor daily body weights as an indication of nutritional and fluid-volume status.
   g) Monitor formula dilution, water supplements, and fluids used to flush tube.
   h) Institute practices that avoid contamination and infection.

1. A client who has hepatitis is receiving IV therapy to correct dehydration secondary to vomiting. The client's vital signs are: blood pressure = 118/64, pulse = 78, respirations = 20. Which of the following IV fluids would be contraindicated for this client?

   a. D_5W (5% dextrose in water)
   b. Normal saline (0.9% NaCl)
   c. Half-strength saline (0.45% NaCl)
   d. Lactated Ringer's

2. An adult client is NPO after abdominal surgery. The surgeon orders 2000 ml of 5% dextrose in 0.45% saline daily. The nurse recognizes that the dextrose in this solution will have which of the following benefits for this client?

   a. It meets the client's nutritional needs until the client can resume oral intake.
   b. It increases osmotic pressure to hold fluid in the vascular space.
   c. It provides sufficient carbohydrate to prevent the ketosis of starvation.
   d. It protects the red blood cells (RBCs) from crenation due to the hypotonic fluid.

3. The physician orders 2000 ml of D_5W to be administered in 24 hours. The IV set has a drop factor of 10 gtt/ml. At what flow rate should the nurse run the IV?

   a. 7 gtt/minute
   b. 12 gtt/minute
   c. 14 gtt/minute
   d. 17 gtt/minute

4. The nurse is assessing a client's peripheral IV site and should recognize which of the following as a sign of infiltration?

   a. Skin around the site feels cooler than the rest of the skin.
   b. IV flow rate becomes faster without adjustment of the roller clamp.
   c. Flow stops when the nurse puts pressure on the vein above the site.
   d. A red streak following the course of the vein appears above the site.

5. A client has a central venous catheter in the subclavian vein. To reduce the client's risk for air embolism, the nurse should:

   a. Place the client in a high Fowler's position during tubing changes.
   b. Change the IV container before the previous container empties.
   c. Ask the client to take deep breaths while the tubing is being changed.
   d. Cover the site with sterile gauze after the central line is removed.

6. A 70-year-old man is severely anemic. Two units of packed red blood cells are ordered for him. While the blood is being administered, the nurse should monitor him closely for:

   a. Jaundice.
   b. Respiratory depression.
   c. Cerebral edema.
   d. Circulatory overload.

7. A client receives 2 units of packed red blood cells and 1 liter of normal saline solution to reverse hypovolemic shock. It will be important to monitor this client for signs of:

   a. Hypercalcemia.
   b. Hypokalemia.
   c. Hypomagnesemia.
   d. Hypochloremia.

8. A client is receiving a standard TPN solution with 25% dextrose. The client has normal liver and kidney functions. When the client's blood glucose becomes elevated, low doses of insulin are started. If none of the electrolytes have been supplemented excessively, this client is at greatest risk for which electrolyte imbalance due to such therapy?

a. Hypokalemia
b. Hyperphosphatemia
c. Hypochloremia
d. Hypermagnesemia

9. An 18-year-old female client has received TPN therapy for 3 months to treat malnutrition due to anorexia nervosa. When she begins oral feedings, she expresses a desire to eat but states that food doesn't taste right and it smells funny. Such symptoms are most likely caused by:

   a. Psychological resistance to eating.
   b. Zinc deficiency.
   c. Hypokalemia.
   d. Effects of dextrose on the hypothalamus.

10. A 70-year-old widower is hospitalized with severe protein-calorie malnutrition. Tube feedings of Osmolite, 1800 ml/day, are initiated. As the client shifts to an anabolic state, he may need which of the following electrolytes supplemented?

    a. Sodium
    b. Calcium
    c. Chloride
    d. Phosphorus

11. An 85-year-old client is receiving tube feedings of Ensure HN at 85 ml/hour to promote healing of a pressure ulcer. The gastrostomy tube is flushed with 30 ml of distilled water every 4 hours. The client's oral mucous membranes are dry and sticky, and the client is restless and disoriented. Which of the following nursing diagnoses is most appropriate for this client?

    a. Alteration in potassium balance (hypokalemia) related to refeeding syndrome
    b. Alteration in sodium balance (hypernatremia) related to hyperosmolar feeding
    c. Alteration in magnesium balance (hypomagnesemia) related to increased protein synthesis
    d. Alteration in calcium balance (hypercalcemia) related to high calcium content of feeding solution

12. A client is receiving a feeding solution that provides 2 kcal/ml via gastrostomy tube with 50-ml flushes every 4 hours. A nursing diagnosis of diarrhea has been made for this client. The most appropriate etiology is:

    a. Administration of hyperosmolar feeding solution.
    b. High fat content of tube-feeding formula.
    c. Excessive fluid intake through frequent tube flushing.
    d. Gastrointestinal irritability caused by the presence of the tube.

ANSWERS

1. **Correct answer is d.** Clients with liver disease should not receive solutions containing lactate. The liver normally converts lactate to bicarbonate. If liver function is impaired, lactate and lactic acid may accumulate.

   a. D_5W is used as a hydrating solution. If the client's blood pressure were low, an electrolyte solution would be preferred.
   b. Normal saline would provide chloride to replace that lost in gastric fluids while the client was vomiting. It would be an appropriate fluid.
   c. Half-strength saline would provide some sodium and chloride to replace losses from vomiting, as well as free water to correct fluid volume deficit.

2. **Correct answer is c.** 2000 ml of a solution containing 5% dextrose provides 100 g of dextrose. This is sufficient to prevent ketosis associated with the metabolic changes caused by starvation.

   a. 100 g of dextrose provides only 340 calories, which would not meet the nutritional needs of an adult.
   b. The opposite is true: Dextrose is rapidly metabolized and the water is free to disperse into all body fluid compartments.

d. Hemolysis of RBCs occurs in hypotonic fluid. Crenation is the shriveling seen when RBCs are exposed to hypertonic solutions.

3. Correct answer is c. The formula is:

$$\frac{2000 \text{ ml} \times 10 \text{ gtt/ml}}{24 \text{ hours} \times 60 \text{ minutes/hour}} = \frac{20,000}{1440} = 13.89$$

Rounding off to the nearest whole number yields a rate of 14 gtt/minute.

a. This would be the correct rate if 1000 ml in 24 hours were ordered.
b. This would be the correct rate if 1700 ml in 24 hours were ordered.
d. This would be the correct rate if 2500 ml in 24 hours were ordered.

4. Correct answer is a. As fluid accumulates due to infiltration, the skin around the site feels significantly cooler than the rest of the skin, because IV fluid is cooler than body temperature.

b. Flow rate decreases when the IV is infusing into the tissue instead of the vein.
c. This indicates that no infiltration has occurred.
d. This is a sign of phlebitis, not infiltration.

5. Correct answer is b. Discontinuing the infusion before the container empties reduces the risk of air entering the IV line. Air in the IV line may be drawn into the vein by the negative pressure in the chest on inspiration.

a. The client should be in Trendelenburg position during tubing changes.
c. The client should perform the Valsalva maneuver while the tubing is changed.
d. Sterile gauze dressing is not occlusive and would therefore be insufficient to prevent air from entering the track left when the catheter is removed. An occlusive dressing is needed.

6. Correct answer is d. Circulatory overload is a frequent complication of blood administration.

a. Jaundice is a sign of hepatitis. It would not occur during the transfusion.

b. Dyspnea, cough, and tachypnea due to fluid overload or wheezing due to anaphylaxis might occur. Respiratory depression is unlikely.
c. Packed RBCs do not contain free water, so they neither lower plasma osmolality nor cause intracellular fluid excess. Cerebral edema would not occur.

7. Correct answer is c. Citrate, the preservative used in stored blood, chelates magnesium, reducing serum magnesium levels. Administration of sodium-rich fluid can increase magnesium excretion.

a. Hypocalcemia may be more likely, because citrate chelates calcium.
b. Hyperkalemia can occur with administration of aged blood, because hemolysis of some RBCs occurs during storage.
d. Trauma and shock can induce sodium and chloride retention. Hyperchloremia may occur with normal saline administration, because it has a higher chloride content than plasma does.

8. Correct answer is a. Although any electrolyte imbalance can occur with TPN, hypokalemia is most likely for this client. Insulin transports potassium into cells, thereby lowering serum levels.

b. Because protein synthesis consumes phosphate, hypophosphatemia is more likely.
c. Standard TPN solutions meet daily requirements of sodium and chloride. Chloride balance is not commonly altered by TPN therapy.
d. Hypomagnesemia may be more likely, as a result of magnesium shifting into cells with TPN therapy.

9. Correct answer is b. Zinc deficiency may occur during prolonged TPN. Alterations in taste and smell are symptoms.

a. Psychologic resistance to eating does not usually produce changes in taste and smell. This client more likely would say she is too full or would express concern about weight gain if this were the problem.

c. Hypokalemia does not produce taste and smell changes.

d. The hypothalamus does not regulate taste and smell. Dextrose would not alter those senses.

10. **Correct answer is d.** Potassium, phosphorus, and magnesium shift into cells as the starved patient shifts to an anabolic state.

    a. If hyponatremia occurs, it is usually due to excess water provided during flushing of the feeding tube. It would be treated by decreasing water intake, not supplementing sodium.
    b and **c.** Abnormalities of calcium and chloride are not usually related to tube feedings.

11. **Correct answer is b.** High-osmolality formulas increase the risk of hypernatremia. IIN stands for high nitrogen, meaning that this is a high-protein formula, which would have a high osmolality. This client is receiving only 180 ml of water daily in flushes, thereby increasing the risk for hypernatremia. Dry mucous membranes, restlessness, and disorientation all are signs of hypernatremia.

    a. Hypokalemia produces muscular weakness, decreased bowel motility, and cardiac irritability.

    c. Hypomagnesemia causes increased deep-tendon reflexes, tremors, tachycardia, and altered mental status.

    d. Hypercalcemia causes behavior changes, muscular weakness, constipation, polyuria, and GI symptoms.

12. **Correct answer is a.** Most feeding products contain 1 kcal/ml. Those that contain 2 kcal/ml have less water content. As these hyperosmolar solutions enter the intestine, the high osmotic pressure draws fluid into the intestine, stimulating peristalsis.

    b. Tube-feeding formulas generally are not high in fat. At least part of their fat content is supplied as medium-chain triglycerides, which do not stimulate diarrhea.
    c. 50-ml flushes every 4 hours provide only 300 ml/day of water, which would not represent excessive intake.
    d. Gastrostomy tubes are secured with retention disks and balloon tips, and they do not cause much irritation of the gastric mucosa.

6

Age-Associated Problems

NURSING HIGHLIGHTS

1. Fluid volume deficiency can occur extremely rapidly in infants and children and can be life threatening; infants and children require more frequent monitoring than do adults.
2. Oral rehydration is always preferred over parenteral rehydration when time and the client's health status permit; most children require assistance and encouragement to consume an adequate amount of rehydration fluids.
3. A gradual decrease in the functioning of major systems, coupled with underlying disease, exacerbates fluid and electrolyte imbalances in the elderly.
4. Many elderly clients suffer from dehydration because fluids are inaccessible to them; the nurse must compensate for a client's physical and mental impairment by making fluids easily and frequently available.
5. Dehydration with hypernatremia is one common cause of mental confusion in the elderly.

fontanel—space in an infant's skull where cranial sutures intersect; covered by tough membranes until calcification is complete

pylorus—muscle at the base of the stomach that controls emptying of the stomach into the small intestine

I. Infants and children

A. Physiologic differences in fluid and electrolyte balance

    1. Differences in fluid volume

        a) Increased percentage of body water: premature (low-birth-weight) newborn 80%–90%, full-term newborn 70%–80%, adult 60%

        b) Large body surface area in relation to weight: increased water lost through skin

        c) Differences in fluid distribution

            (1) Newborn extracellular fluid (ECF) is 40% of body weight; at age 1, ECF is 30%; adult ECF is 20%.

See text pages
_____

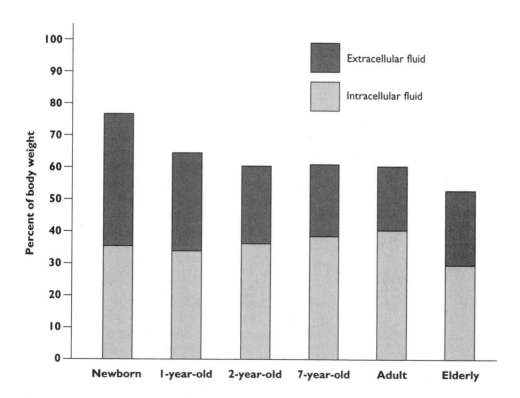

Figure 6–1
Age-Related Changes in Total Body Fluids and Fluid Distribution

(2) Newborn intracellular fluid (ICF) is 30%–40% of body weight; at age 1, ICF is 34%; adult ICF is 40%.

(3) Higher ratio of ECF to ICF predisposes infant to more rapid fluid loss; ratio remains high until child reaches age 3–5.

d) Higher fluid turnover in infant: An infant uses and replaces about half of the ECF daily, whereas an adult uses and replaces about a sixth.

2. Immature renal mechanisms

a) Kidneys unable to fully concentrate urine until age 2; high volume of urine relative to size of child

b) Low glomerular filtration rate; excess fluid not effectively excreted

3. Less effective acid-base homeostasis

a) Lower acid-base buffering capacity

b) Higher metabolic rate: more metabolic wastes produced

4. Immature endocrine system

a) Poor response to excess phosphates and sulfates (e.g., from cow's milk)

b) Immature response aggravated by illness, vitamin D deficiency

B. Normal laboratory values in children

1. Serum sodium: infant 139–146 mg/L; child 138–145 mg/L

2. Serum potassium: infant 4.1–5.3 mg/L; child 3.4–4.7 mg/L

3. Serum calcium: newborn 9.0–10.6 mg/dl; infant 9.6–9.8 mg/dl; child 8.8–10.8 mg/dl

4. Serum chloride: infant 96–116 mEq/L; child 90–110 mEq/L

5. Serum magnesium: infant 1.4–1.9 mg/dl; child 1.4–1.7 mg/dl

6. Blood urea nitrogen: 10–25 mg/dl

7. Creatinine: 0.7–1.4 mg/dl

8. Hemoglobin: 11.5–15.5 g/dl

9. Hematocrit: 35%–45%

10. pH: newborn 7.27–7.47; child 7.33–7.43

11. $PaCO_2$ (partial pressure of carbon dioxide in arterial blood): newborn 27–40 mm Hg; infant 27–41 mm Hg; child and adult 35–45 mm Hg

12. HCO_3 (bicarbonate): newborn 22–30 mEq/L; child and adult 22–26 mEq/L

C. Conditions creating fluid and electrolyte imbalances

1. Diarrhea

a) Diarrhea with isotonic dehydration, or iso-osmolar fluid volume deficit (FVD): sodium and water lost in equal amounts; ECF decreased; occurs in 70% of clients with severe diarrhea

(1) Pathophysiology and etiology: No osmotic pull from ICF to ECF; plasma volume reduced; diarrhea, vomiting, and malnutrition

(2) Signs and symptoms: hypovolemic shock (see Chapter 2, section I,C, for additional discussion); notable signs in children include rapid weight loss, sunken eyeballs, sunken anterior fontanel, absence of tearing, and irritability; serum sodium 130–150 mEq/L

(3) Treatment and management: Restore fluid volume with iso-osmolar fluids IV or PO; reduce diarrhea and vomiting with appropriate diet.

b) Diarrhea with hypertonic dehydration, or hyperosmolar FVD: water loss greater than sodium loss (hypernatremia); occurs in 20% of clients with severe diarrhea

(1) Pathophysiology and etiology: ICF loss; increased osmolality of ECF draws fluid from cells; severe diarrhea or restricted water intake or both; fever; and poor renal function

(2) Signs and symptoms: thirst, weight loss, confusion, convulsions, thickened and firm skin turgor, decreased urine output, brain injury, and hypernatremia (see Chapter 3, section II,C); shock less apparent than in iso-osmolar dehydration; blood pressure in children often normal; serum sodium greater than 150 mEq/L

(3) Treatment and management: Increase ICF and ECF with 5% dextrose in 0.2% sodium chloride (NaCl) or similar solution; watch for signs of water intoxication; avoid large quantities of 5% dextrose in water (D_5W).

c) Diarrhea with hypotonic dehydration, or hypo-osmolar FVD: sodium loss in excess of fluids (hyponatremia); ECF is decreased and ICF is increased; found in 10% of clients with severe diarrhea

(1) Pathophysiology and etiology: higher osmolality of ICF draws water into cell, depleting ECF; severe diarrhea, cholera, and bacillary dysentery; excessive infusion of D_5W; sodium-wasting diuretics and sodium-wasting renal disease

(2) Signs and symptoms: shock symptoms; decreased urine output, thirst, weight loss, lethargy, coma, poor skin turgor, clammy skin, and soft eyeballs; serum sodium less than 130 mEq/L

(3) Treatment and management: Rehydrate using lactated Ringer's, 5% dextrose in 0.45% NaCl, or equivalent solutions; rapid infusion may cause overhydration and congestive heart failure.

2. Pyloric stenosis: affects 1 of every 750 female and 1 of every 150 male infants; pylorus is elongated, producing a narrowed outlet from stomach to duodenum

a) Pathophysiology and etiology: repeated vomiting; infant unable to retain adequate nutrition; causes FVD with metabolic alkalosis, potassium deficit, and sodium deficit

b) Signs and symptoms: projectile vomiting after each feeding; fluid volume deficit; decreased respiration and other signs of respiratory alkalosis (see Chapter 4, section V,B), palpable pyloric mass, and ketoacidosis in prolonged starvation

        c) Treatment and management: IV therapy to restore fluid and electrolyte balance, then corrective surgery

   3. Excessive water intake: water intoxication; infant capacity to excrete excess fluids limited by low glomerular filtration rate

        a) Pathophysiology and etiology: free water accumulates in extracellular space, producing hyponatremia; excessive dilution of formula; swallowing large amount of water when swimming; tap water enemas; inappropriate oral or IV rehydration of dehydrated infant

        b) Signs and symptoms: pulmonary and cerebral edema, lethargy, irritability, subnormal temperature, seizures, and respiratory distress

        c) Treatment and management: Restrict free water; elevate serum sodium.

   4. Constipation: fluid and electrolyte imbalance caused by use of enemas; hyperphosphatemia, hypocalcemia, or hypernatremia; use iso-osmolar saline for enema

   5. Others: Conditions that cause electrolyte imbalances in adults also cause them in children: surgery, burns (see Chapter 7, section IV), renal disease (see Chapter 10), syndrome of inappropriate antidiuretic hormone, and diabetic ketoacidosis (see Chapter 12).

D. Signs and symptoms: general considerations concerning the young

   1. Fluids and electrolyte imbalances occur much more rapidly in infants and children than in adults.

   2. Dehydration is very common in infants and children.

        a) Mild: loss of 2%–5% of body weight; heart rate elevated 10%–15% above baseline; dry mucous membranes, concentrated urine, and reduced tearing

        b) Moderate: loss of 6%–9% of body weight; increased severity of mild symptoms; reduced urine output, decreased skin turgor, and sunken eyeballs and anterior fontanel

        c) Severe: loss of 10% or more of body weight; extremely increased severity of moderate symptoms; decreased blood pressure, no urine output, and metabolic acidosis

   3. Skin turgor is not a reliable sign of dehydration in plump infants and children or in cases of hyperosmolar dehydration.

   4. Blood pressure may remain normal in children with fluid volume deficit because of elasticity of young arteries.

   5. Additional electrolyte imbalances (e.g., hypokalemia, hypomagnesemia, metabolic alkalosis, metabolic acidosis) can occur secondary to primary imbalance due to vomiting, diarrhea, and changes in fluid distribution.

E. Treatment and management: general considerations concerning the young
   1. Primary goal is to restore fluid and electrolyte imbalance; secondary goal is to stop vomiting or diarrhea or both or correct underlying cause of imbalance.
      a) Volume of replacement fluids depends on the weight of the child.
         (1) 100 ml/kg for first 10 kg of body weight
         (2) 50 ml/kg for next 10 kg of body weight
         (3) 20 ml/kg for each kg more than 20 kg of body weight
      b) Additional factors such as fever, renal abnormalities, and high environmental temperature may necessitate deviation from formula.
   2. Oral rehydration is preferred over parenteral rehydration when time and the client's condition permit.
   3. Commercially available fluids provide balanced replacement of sodium, potassium, chloride, bicarbonate, and glucose for oral rehydration (e.g., oral rehydration solution [ORS], Infalyte, Lytren, Pedialyte, Rehydralyte, Resol); other fluids (e.g., fruit juice, sodas) provide partial replacement.
   4. Parenteral replacement fluid must be infused slowly to prevent overhydration; oral replacement fluids must be offered frequently and in small amounts.
   5. Specific treatment and management of common fluid volume and electrolyte imbalances can be found in Chapters 2 and 3 and apply to children as well as adults.

F. Nursing process: special concerns in children and infants (for a discussion of the general nursing process for all clients with fluid imbalances, see Chapter 2, sections I,E and II,E)
   1. Nursing assessment
      a) Obtain child's health history from parents, keeping in mind that parents may have difficulty estimating the frequency and quantities of fluids the child lost.
      b) Assess child's baseline vital signs; reassess as needed, sometimes as frequently as every 15 minutes for seriously ill child.
      c) Weigh child to obtain a baseline weight; if child's preillness weight is known, compare weights for signs of dehydration.
      d) Obtain baseline values for laboratory tests, and evaluate based on a knowledge of the normal values for the age of the child.
      e) Assess child for signs of fluid volume and electrolyte imbalances, paying special attention to absence of tears, dry mucous membranes, skin turgor, and chest sounds.
      f) Assess neurologic signs.
   2. Nursing diagnoses common in infants and children
      a) Fluid volume deficit related to vomiting, diarrhea, and/or decreased fluid intake
      b) Altered bowel elimination, diarrhea, related to irritable bowel
      c) Impaired skin integrity related to destruction of skin secondary to edema or diarrhea

I. Infants and children	II. The elderly client	III. Pregnancy

d) Altered nutrition, less than body requirements, related to anorexia secondary to nausea, vomiting, and/or diarrhea

e) Fluid volume excess related to inadequate excretion of urine, excessive rehydration, or overly rapid rehydration

3. Nursing interventions for infants and children

a) Monitor vital signs, laboratory tests, and neurologic signs frequently, because fluid volume imbalances can occur rapidly in infants and children.

b) Identify source of fluid volume imbalance.

c) Accurately record child's fluid intake and output, including vomitus and loose stools.

d) Monitor changes in child's weight.

e) Take steps to alleviate cause of fluid imbalance (e.g., alter diet to reduce diarrhea or vomiting).

f) When oral rehydration is possible, offer small sips of fluids frequently, providing as much physical assistance as needed (e.g., holding cup).

g) Educate parents concerning home care of child with diarrhea and signs and symptoms of fluid imbalances (see Client Teaching Checklist, "Diarrhea in Infants and Children").

✔ CLIENT TEACHING CHECKLIST ✔

Diarrhea in Infants and Children

Serious dehydration can develop rapidly in infants and children. Give the following information to parents.

✔ Children have low fluid reserves and need replacement fluids immediately.

✔ Children with fever need extra replacement fluids.

✔ Children better tolerate small amounts of liquids given frequently rather than large amounts given occasionally.

✔ Children's preferences in fluids should be considered; Popsicles and ice are good sources of fluids.

✔ Milk is not tolerated well by children who are vomiting.

✔ The BRAT (banana, rice, applesauce, toast) diet is most easily tolerated by children recovering from diarrhea.

✔ Balanced replacement fluids (e.g., Infalyte, Pedialyte) are available at pharmacies and without a prescription.

✔ Seek medical help immediately if the child is not urinating, has a high fever, appears lethargic, produces no tears when crying, or in other ways behaves abnormally.

h) Explain to child—at child's level of understanding—the need for oral or IV rehydration therapy.

i) Provide care for compromised tissue (e.g., clean skin, change diaper often); involve parents when possible.

II. The elderly client: Underlying disease often aggravates imbalances.

See text pages _____

A. Physiologic differences in fluid and electrolyte balance: more difficulty maintaining fluid and electrolyte homeostasis complicated by diminished function of major systems; slower adaptation to fluid and electrolyte changes

1. Changes in fluid distribution: total body water decreased to about 46%–52% of body weight; decreased ratio of ICF to ECF; predisposes to fluid volume deficit

2. Renal changes
   a) Decreased number of functioning nephrons beginning at age 40, reduced by 30%–50% by age 70, with thickening of glomerular membranes; reduced ability to concentrate urine
   b) Decreased glomerular filtration rate (by 46% between the ages of 20 and 90); increased solute load and accumulation of wastes

3. Pulmonary changes
   a) Decreased elasticity of lung tissue and fewer alveoli; defective alveolar ventilation
   b) Decreased strength of chest muscles: chest wall more rigid, accumulation of bronchial secretions and carbon dioxide retention, difficulty regulating pH

4. Cardiovascular changes
   a) Decreased elasticity of blood vessel walls: arteriosclerosis; increased blood pressure in capillaries; fluid moves into tissues, causing edema
   b) Decreased stroke volume and cardiac output (1% per year from ages 20 to 80): blood flow decreased; cardiac reserve decreased; heart adapts more slowly to increased demands
   c) Decreased sensitivity of baroreceptor: reduced ability to compensate for hypotensive shock

5. Gastrointestinal changes
   a) Decreased volume of gastric juice: predisposes to hypokalemia, hyponatremia, and metabolic alkalosis during vomiting or gastric suction
   b) Decreased calcium absorption: predisposes to hypocalcemia or osteoporosis
   c) Decreased volume of saliva: dry mouth
   d) Decreased gastrointestinal motility: predisposes to constipation and may promote laxative abuse (see this chapter, section II,B,4)

6. Changes in regulatory functions
   a) Liver cells decrease in size: decreased capacity to detoxify drugs
   b) Decreased glucose tolerance: predisposes to hyperglycemia and fluid volume deficit

          c) Decreased secretion of aldosterone: reduced capacity to conserve sodium and excrete potassium

          d) Decreased response of distal tubules of kidney to vasopressin and decreased ability to make and excrete ammonia: predispose to metabolic acid-base imbalances

          e) Decreased sensation of thirst: predisposes to fluid volume deficit

      7. Skin changes

          a) Thinning and decreased elasticity of skin; skin turgor no longer good indicator of hydration status

          b) Decreased blood flow and decreased functional sweat glands; reduced ability to maintain body temperatures

B. Special problems of fluid and electrolyte imbalances

    1. Dehydration: decreased ECF volume

        a) Pathophysiology and etiology

           (1) Decreased fluid intake: sensitivity of thirst receptors diminished, reduced access to fluids (common in mobility-impaired clients in nursing homes), physical problems with swallowing, mental confusion, and tube feeding

           (2) Increased fluid loss: diarrhea, vomiting, fever, and renal disease

        b) Signs and symptoms (see Chapter 2, section I,C, for signs and symptoms common to all ages)

           (1) Skin turgor is not a reliable sign in an elderly client, as skin elasticity is lost with increasing age.

           (2) Hypernatremia often occurs with FVD in the elderly, adding to mental confusion.

        c) Treatment and management: Restore fluid volume either PO or IV; treat underlying cause; provide assistance for mobility-impaired clients.

    2. Edema: increased ECF volume

        a) Pathophysiology and etiology: overhydration from IV therapy, increased capillary pressure from arteriosclerosis, renal failure, and cardiac insufficiency

        b) Signs and symptoms (see Chapter 2, section II,C)

        c) Treatment and management: Reduce free water cautiously; treat underlying disease; use diuretics with great caution.

    3. Problems arising from diuretic use

        a) Thiazide diuretics and furosemide (e.g., Lasix), used to treat congestive heart failure and hypertension, are potassium wasting.

           (1) The elderly are especially susceptible to hypokalemia induced by diuretics.

   (2) Hypokalemia potentiates the action of digitalis, predisposing to toxic shock.

  b) Potassium-sparing diuretics such as spironolactone (e.g., Aldactone) or triamterene (e.g., Dyrenium) may cause hyperkalemia in the elderly.

  c) Thiazide diuretics may cause hyponatremia in the elderly.

  d) All diuretics may cause FVD; resulting dizziness predisposes the elderly to falls.

4. Problems arising from laxative abuse
  a) Predisposes to FVD and hypokalemia
  b) Predisposes to diarrhea: Elderly clients have reduced ability to metabolize drugs; gradual buildup of active ingredients (e.g., phenolphthalein) can result in excessive effects.

5. Problems arising from antacid use
  a) Antacids containing calcium carbonate or aluminum hydroxide often cause constipation, resulting in dependency on laxatives.
  b) Increased use of antacids containing bicarbonate may predispose to metabolic alkalosis.

6. Preparation for diagnostic tests: colon cleansing
  a) Fluid restrictions before test stress limited fluid reserves of the elderly.
  b) Purgatives (e.g., castor oil, magnesium citrate, bisacodyl [Dulcolax]) remove large amounts of fluids and electrolytes; resulting fluid shifts among body compartments can be dangerous when cardiovascular disease is present.
  c) Radiocontrast media increase solute load; response is limited by age-related loss of renal function, and resulting osmotic diuresis can exacerbate fluid loss.

7. Osteoporosis: bone thinning due to inadequate total body calcium; increased incidence of fractures; common in postmenopausal women, most frequent in small-boned white women older than age 50
  a) Laboratory findings: Serum concentrations of calcium and phosphate are normal, but deficits exist in total body calcium and phosphate.
  b) Pathophysiology and etiology: decreased calcium intake, decreased physical activity, impaired calcium absorption, increased parathyroid hormone, and reduced estrogen secretion; bone mass lost as calcium is ionized
  c) Treatment and management: combination of oral calcium supplements (minimum 1000 mg/day), vitamin D (minimum 400 IU/day), and estrogen (may cause side effects, including sodium retention and hypertension); exercise program appropriate to general health, abilities, and lifestyle (exercise, especially weight-bearing activities, can increase bone mass)

8. Hyperthermia: heatstroke; clients older than age 70 most severely affected (see Nurse Alert, "Diagnosing Heat Stress in the Elderly")
  a) Pathophysiology and etiology: altered sweating mechanism reduces heat loss from skin; decreased perception of warmth;

reduced cardiac response to heat stress; use of medications (e.g., diuretics) that alter thermoregulation

   b) Treatment and management: Reduce environmental temperatures; encourage fluid consumption; reduce physical activity.

9. Perioperative concerns: major surgery tolerated less well by the elderly; cardiac and pulmonary complications common; good preoperative preparation saves lives

   a) Restriction of oral fluid intake before surgery predisposes to fluid volume deficit; start IV fluids before surgery.

   b) Infusions of cool fluids and cool temperatures in operating room predispose to hypothermia; keep client warm.

   c) Decreased respiratory function promotes respiratory acidosis; keep airways clear, and change client's position as frequently as possible.

   d) Electrolyte and pH imbalances are poorly tolerated; detect and correct before surgery.

10. Hyperosmolar hyperglycemic nonketotic (HHNK) coma: commonly caused by mild, undiagnosed diabetes in the elderly (see Chapter 12 for a discussion of HHNK coma)

C. Nursing process

1. Nursing assessment: special concerns in the elderly (for a discussion of the general nursing process for all clients with fluid imbalances, see Chapter 2, sections I,E, II,E, and III,E)

   a) Obtain client's medical history, keeping in mind that client may be confused or forget about some medications.

   b) Obtain client's baseline vital signs, keeping in mind that body temperature decreases with age.

! NURSE *ALERT* !

Diagnosing Heat Stress in the Elderly

The elderly are more prone to heat stress because of age-related impairments in thermoregulation. Normal body temperature decreases significantly with age and may be close to 97°F (36.1°C) in the elderly. An elderly client with a body temperature of 99°F (37.2°C) may be experiencing heat stress despite the seemingly mild temperature elevation.

c) Obtain client's baseline laboratory test values.

d) Determine client's baseline weight.

e) Assess client for fluid volume imbalances, using hand- and foot-vein filling rather than skin turgor.

f) Assess client's ability to obtain fluids independently (e.g., ambulation, use of hands).

g) Assess the effect of age-related physiologic changes and underlying disease on fluid-volume and health status.

2. Nursing diagnoses common in the elderly

a) Fluid volume deficit related to decreased fluid intake (very common)

b) Fluid volume excess, edema, secondary to cardiac insufficiency

c) Alternate bowel elimination, constipation, related to decreased fluid intake, decreased gastrointestinal motility, and/or laxative abuse

d) Increased body temperature, heat stress, related to decreased sweating and inadequate fluid intake

3. Nursing interventions for the elderly

a) Monitor client's baseline vital signs, changes in weight, and changes in laboratory test results.

b) Assist physically or mentally impaired clients in obtaining adequate fluids; educate families and caregivers on the need to make fluids easily and frequently available.

c) Encourage clients to exercise (mildly), ambulate, or change positions in bed to promote better respiration and bone mass maintenance.

d) Educate clients and their families on the appropriate use of laxatives, diuretics, and antacids.

e) Monitor client's nutritional status, with emphasis on protein and calcium intake.

f) Monitor client's fluid intake and output.

g) Treat client's underlying conditions, as directed by a physician.

h) Provide IV fluids preoperatively and postoperatively as directed.

i) Respond to changes in environmental temperature by adjusting client's clothing, bedding, and fluid intake as appropriate for comfort.

III. Pregnancy: a condition of health causing fluid and electrolyte changes

See text pages
_____

A. Normal fluid and electrolyte changes: Values return to prepregnancy levels shortly after delivery and without intervention.

1. Increased blood volume: nearly 50% plasma volume increase (more if twins); results in decreased hematocrit and hemoglobin values

2. Increased fluid retention: increased retention of about 950 mEq sodium and 7 liters of water

            a) Edema: occurs in the absence of hypertension in up to 85% of pregnancies; dependent or generalized

            b) Plasma sodium concentration: falls about 5 mEq/L during first 2 months in response to increased antidiuretic hormone and water retention

       3. Calcium balance: begins falling at end of first trimester; calcium needed for fetal skeleton

       4. Other electrolytes: magnesium falls 6%–9% as an artifact of increased plasma volume; 350 mEq potassium cumulatively retained

       5. Acid-base changes: Compensated respiratory alkalosis due to stimulation of the respiratory center of the medulla by progesterone; serum bicarbonate drops (compensation)

   B. Complications of pregnancy causing fluid and electrolyte changes

       1. Pregnancy-induced hypertension (i.e., preeclampsia, formerly toxemia): develops in 5%–7% of pregnancies in about week 20 of pregnancy; most at-risk women younger than 20 or older than 35 years; etiology unknown; third-leading cause of maternal death in United States

       2. Hyponatremia induced by oxytocin administration: Labor induction with oxytocin (an antidiuretic) infused in large amounts of D_5W can produce water intoxication seizures in woman and fetus; use a balanced electrolyte solution (e.g., normal saline or lactated Ringer's) in place of D_5W, and limit fluid intake.

1. The best site for assessing skin turgor on a 2-year-old of normal weight is the:
   a. Anterior scalp.
   b. Dorsum of the hand.
   c. Scapula.
   d. Medial thigh.

2. When a child younger than 2 years of age requires an enema, the nurse should anticipate that which of the following solutions will be ordered?
   a. Soap and water
   b. Tap water
   c. Normal saline
   d. Sodium phosphate (Fleet)

3. A client reports feeding cow's milk to a 6-month-old infant. The nurse should explain that cow's milk should not be fed to infants because:
   a. It provides inadequate calcium for bone growth.
   b. The high sodium content of cow's milk can lead to brain injury.
   c. It does not contain enough water to meet infants' fluid needs.
   d. It provides excess phosphorus, which can damage kidneys and joints.

4. A 4-year-old is recovering from diarrhea. Which of the following snacks would be appropriate for this client?
   a. Half of a banana
   b. Oatmeal with milk
   c. Orange sections
   d. Mashed carrots

5. A 75-year-old client reports daily use of a phenolphthalein laxative to prevent constipation. It is most important that the nurse assess this client for a deficit of:
   a. Potassium.
   b. Sodium.
   c. Calcium.
   d. Chloride.

6. An 80-year-old client has dehydration and hypernatremia. Which of the following nursing diagnoses is most likely to apply to this client?
   a. Alteration in nutrition related to anorexia and nausea
   b. Urine retention related to renal conservation of fluid
   c. Alteration in thought processes related to inadequate fluid intake
   d. Alteration in comfort related to paresthesias of the hands and face

7. A 70-year-old woman has osteoporosis. Calcium supplements are prescribed for her. Which of the following nursing measures would increase the effectiveness of those supplements in reducing her bone loss?
   a. Encouraging her to increase her fluid intake
   b. Assisting her to walk the length of the hallway
   c. Suggesting she consult her gynecologist about discontinuing her estrogen supplements
   d. Cautioning her to avoid exposure to direct sunlight

8. The nurse has identified that a client is at high risk for heat stress during a heat wave. The nurse should teach the client to:
   a. Eat more protein and less carbohydrate during the heat wave.
   b. Wear clothing made of lightweight, synthetic fabric.
   c. Take the walk that is part of the daily routine in the early morning.
   d. Avoid sitting directly in the flow of air from the living room fan.

9. A 31-year-old woman in her second trimester of pregnancy complains of swelling of her ankles and feet. To reduce her discomfort, the nurse should teach her to:

a. Rest in a side-lying position several times a day.
b. Wear a maternity girdle to support the abdomen.
c. Limit fluid intake to 5–6 glasses per day.
d. Increase intake of sodium-rich foods.

10. When evaluating the acid-base balance of a pregnant woman, the nurse should expect to find compensated:
a. Respiratory acidosis.
b. Respiratory alkalosis.
c. Metabolic acidosis.
d. Metabolic alkalosis.

11. A woman who is 38 weeks pregnant has developed preeclampsia and is oliguric. The nurse should question an order for which of the following IV fluids?
a. Normal saline solution
b. Ringer's solution
c. 5% albumin solution
d. D_5W

12. A woman who has pregnancy-induced hypertension develops eclampsia. She is receiving IV magnesium sulfate. Which of the following assessments should be reported to the physician immediately?
a. Pedal edema, 2+
b. Absence of the patellar reflex
c. Urinary output >100 ml/hour
d. Hyperventilation

ANSWERS

1. **Correct answer is d.** The abdomen and the medial aspect of the thigh are the best locations to test skin turgor in the child. Tenting is most apparent in those sites when there is a fluid volume deficit.

a, b, and c. Changes in skin turgor at these sites occur later and are not observed as reliably in a child.

2. **Correct answer is c.** Normal saline is the most appropriate solution for enemas administered to young children. It is least likely to significantly alter fluid and electrolyte balance.

a and b. Water should not be used in enemas given to young children. Large amounts of water absorbed from the colon may cause dilutional hyponatremia, with seizures and respiratory distress.
d. Sodium phosphate enemas can cause hyperphosphatemia, hypocalcemia, and hypernatremia in children. Fleet enemas are contraindicated in children under 2 years of age.

3. **Correct answer is d.** Cow's milk provides about 950 mg of phosphorus per liter. Human milk and formulas patterned on it contain only about 150 mg of phosphorus per liter. Hyperphosphatemia may occur in infants fed cow's milk, producing calcification in kidneys, joints, arteries, and corneas.

a. Cow's milk contains more calcium than human milk or formula, although the lower calcium-phosphorus ratio causes infants' immature kidneys to excrete calcium.
b. Shrinking of the brain due to hypernatremia can result in rupture of small blood vessels. However, the sodium content of cow's milk is not sufficiently different from human milk to cause hypernatremia.
c. The water content in cow's milk is adequate to meet fluid needs. It is the electrolyte content that is of concern.

4. **Correct answer is a.** The foods that are best tolerated by the child recovering from diarrhea are represented by the acronym *BRAT*. They are banana, rice, applesauce, and toast.

b. Milk is often not tolerated well by the child who is recovering from vomiting or diarrhea.
c and d. Foods offered to the child recovering from diarrhea should be bland, easy to digest, and low in residue. Neither oranges nor carrots would be good choices; oranges are acidic, and both oranges and carrots are high in fiber.

5. **Correct answer is a.** Phenolphthalein laxatives often have prolonged effects in the elderly, causing frequent and watery stools. Potassium is lost in diarrhea. Because potassium is not stored in the body, the losses are not replaced and a deficit will appear.

b and **d.** Sodium and chloride tend to become decreased when gastric fluid is lost, as in gastric suctioning or vomiting. Some sodium is also lost in loose stools, but it tends to be adequately replaced by dietary intake.

c. If the client's diarrhea were due to a malabsorption syndrome, hypocalcemia would be more likely. If the serum calcium decreases, calcium stored in the bones will be released to replace it, so hypocalcemia is less likely than hypokalemia.

6. **Correct answer is c.** Hypernatremia associated with inadequate oral fluid intake is one of the most common causes of acute confusion in the elderly. Correction of fluid and electrolyte balance often improves the mental status.

a. Anorexia and nausea are signs and symptoms of hyponatremia. Weight loss associated with dehydration is generally due to fluid loss, not inadequate food intake.

b. This client is likely to have a reduced urine output, because the kidneys will conserve fluid. The reduced output is due to decreased urine production, not urine retention.

d. Paresthesias do not represent a common symptom of either dehydration or hypernatremia. They occur more often with imbalances of potassium or calcium.

7. **Correct answer is b.** Exercise, especially weight-bearing exercise, promotes the deposition of calcium in bones. It will, therefore, enhance the effectiveness of the supplements.

a. Increased fluid intake helps reduce the risk of kidney stones when excess calcium is being excreted in urine. It does not promote calcium deposition in bones.

c. Estrogen promotes deposition of calcium in bones. Discontinuing the estrogen would reduce the effectiveness of the calcium supplements.

d. Exposure of the skin to sunlight triggers the synthesis of vitamin D, which promotes calcium absorption and bone formation. Unless contraindicated for other reasons, the client should have some sun exposure; if she does not, she may need vitamin D supplements as well as calcium supplements.

8. **Correct answer is c.** The elderly should avoid exercising during the warmest part of the day. Walking has important benefits, but the client should adjust the routine to perform such exercise during the coolest part of the day, which is early morning.

a. The client should eat more carbohydrate and less protein to decrease the body's heat production due to digestive processes.

b. Light-colored cotton clothing is best. Synthetic fabrics are less absorbent and may retain heat.

d. Moving air promotes evaporation of perspiration, helping to cool the body. During a heat wave, this may be beneficial.

9. **Correct answer is a.** The pressure of the pregnant uterus on the inferior vena cava is a major contributing factor to dependent edema. The side-lying position reduces the pressure of the uterus on the vena cava.

b. Girdles should be avoided because they cause constriction in the abdomen and groin area. Support hose are a better option, because they counteract increased venous hydrostatic pressure.

c. The client needs 8–10 glasses of fluid daily to maintain the expanded maternal extracellular fluid volume. Pedal edema is an expected discomfort, not a symptom of complications.

d. Even though sodium restriction is no longer recommended, moderation is appropriate. High dietary sodium levels would worsen the edema.

10. **Correct answer is b.** Progesterone has a potent stimulant effect on the respiratory center, leading to hyperventilation. Prolonged hyperventilation causes respiratory alkalosis, for which the kidneys compensate by excreting bicarbonate.

a. Respiratory acidosis would be abnormal, suggesting respiratory disease or hypoventilation.
c. Metabolic acidosis would be abnormal, suggesting diabetic ketoacidosis, lactic acidosis, or renal insufficiency.
d. Metabolic alkalosis is abnormal. It may occur as a result of excessive vomiting.

11. **Correct answer is d.** The nurse questions an order that is inappropriate. Hypotonic fluids are contraindicated in preeclampsia, because they may reduce serum osmolality enough to cause cerebral edema.

a and **b.** Isotonic electrolyte solutions are appropriate. They do not alter serum osmolality.

c. Colloids may be used, especially if the serum albumin is low, causing decreased colloid oncotic pressure.

12. **Correct answer is b.** Hypermagnesemia causes loss of deep-tendon reflexes, progressing to respiratory and cardiac depression. The IV magnesium must be discontinued.

a. Pedal edema is a common problem in pregnancy. Edema of the hands or face may appear in pregnancy-induced hypertension. Such an assessment would not, however, indicate an emergency situation.
c. Urinary output should be >100 ml/hour to ensure adequate magnesium excretion. A lower urinary output should be reported.
d. Respiratory depression is a sign of excessive magnesium. Hyperventilation is unlikely to be related to administration of magnesium sulfate.

7

Trauma, Shock, and Burns

NURSING HIGHLIGHTS

1. Hypovolemia can occur with shock or trauma without external blood loss as a result of third-space fluid shifts or venous pooling of blood; normal blood volume becomes unavailable for vascular functions.
2. Behavioral changes are often the first signs of shock; restlessness, irritability, and excitability often occur before changes in vital signs are detected.
3. Many of the signs of shock, trauma, smoke poisoning, and burns do not appear until hours or days later, making reassessment a critical nursing function.
4. Shock, trauma, and burn injuries all are aggravated by preexisting medical conditions, fractures, and either extreme youth or extreme age of the client.

GLOSSARY

vasopressor—a substance given to constrict the blood vessels in the hope of improving blood circulation; examples include: levarterenol bitartrate (Levophed), metaraminol bitartrate (Aramine), dopamine hydrochloride (Intropin, Revimine)

ENHANCED OUTLINE

See text pages

I. General trauma: acute injury; rapid fluid, electrolyte, and acid-base changes

A. Pathophysiology: cellular breakdown
1. Electrolyte changes
a) Potassium leaves cells as they break down, raising serum potassium levels.
b) Sodium and chloride move into cells, causing hyponatremia.
c) Sodium-potassium pump breaks down.
2. Fluid changes
a) Water follows sodium into cells.
b) Fluid shifts into interstitial space at injured site (third-space shift); fluid becomes unavailable for vascular functions, and hypovolemia ensues.
3. Acid-base changes
a) Nonvolatile acids (e.g., lactic acid) are released from cells, causing metabolic acidosis.
b) Decreased removal of hydrogen ions by the kidneys can cause metabolic acidosis.
c) Lungs compensate for metabolic acidosis by hyperventilation.
4. Protein changes
a) Nitrogen is lost due to cell breakdown and reduced protein anabolism.
b) Protein shifts with water to interstitial space.
c) Plasma colloidal osmotic pressure falls while tissue colloidal osmotic pressure rises.
5. Capillary changes: Increased capillary permeability results in fluid loss from vascular space, contributing to hypovolemia.
6. Hormonal influences
a) Hypovolemia stimulates antidiuretic hormone (ADH) production, causing increased water resorption from kidneys.

        b) Syndrome of inappropriate ADH (SIADH) may occur in response to surgery, trauma, and pain, resulting in excess water retention.

        c) Aldosterone is produced in response to hyponatremia and stress, resulting in increased sodium resorption and potassium excretion.

    7. Renal factors: Hypovolemia can cause temporary or permanent kidney damage predisposing to hyperkalemia.

B. Signs and symptoms

    1. Changes in vital signs

        a) Pulse: rate increased above 120 (hypovolemia); full, bounding pulse (hypervolemia); irregular pulse (hypokalemia)

        b) Blood pressure: changes may not occur until hypovolemia is established; systolic pressure drop (hypovolemia); pulse pressure less than 20 mm Hg (shock)

        c) Respiration: rate increased above 32 breaths/minute (hypovolemia); Kussmaul breathing (metabolic acidosis from cell damage); hyperventilation (anxiety or hypoxia)

        d) Temperature: changes often occur hours or days later in the form of mild elevation (hypovolemia or imminent shock) or severe elevation (infection)

    2. Behavioral changes: irritability, apprehension, confusion, or restlessness (hypoxia early; fluid and electrolyte imbalances later)

    3. Neurologic changes: muscular weakness or abdominal distension (hypokalemia, often delayed); confusion, coma (fluid imbalances); twitching or tremors (hypocalcemia or hypomagnesemia or both)

    4. Urinary changes: decreased urine output (hypovolemia, lack of fluid intake)

    5. Circulatory changes: hand and neck veins remain flat (hypovolemia); vein engorgement (overhydration); chest rales (overhydration)

    6. Skin changes

        a) Color: pale, gray (hypovolemia or shock); flushed (hypernatremia or metabolic alkalosis)

        b) Turgor: poor (hypovolemia; may be delayed 1–3 days)

        c) Edema: sodium and water retention

        d) Mucous membranes: dry, sticky (dehydration; may be delayed 1–3 days)

        e) Other: wound draining, increased insensible loss from skin

    7. Laboratory test changes

        a) Electrolytes: may be increased or decreased

        b) Serum carbon dioxide content: decreased (metabolic acidosis); increased (metabolic alkalosis)

        c) Blood urea nitrogen (BUN): increased (dehydration or impaired renal function)

        d) Serum creatinine: increased (impaired renal function)

        e) Arterial blood gases: pH and bicarbonate (HCO_3) decreased (metabolic acidosis)

        f) Hematocrit and hemoglobin: increased (hypovolemia)

g) Electrocardiogram: T wave flat or inverted (cardiac ischemia or hypokalemia or both); T wave peaked (hyperkalemia)

C. Nursing assessment: Assessment must be repeated frequently, as some signs appear only after hours or days.
   1. Assess vital signs, and determine baseline values.
   2. Obtain laboratory test results to establish baseline values.
   3. Obtain client history, with emphasis on drugs influencing fluid and electrolyte imbalances (e.g., potassium-wasting diuretics with digitalis, cortisone, antibiotics).
   4. Evaluate client's sensorium, and assess for neurologic and neuromuscular changes.
   5. Assess for fluid losses.
   6. Assess for signs and symptoms of general trauma and associated fluid and electrolyte imbalances.

See text pages

II. Head injuries: Any increase in brain size causes significant increase in intracranial pressure (ICP) due to nonexpandable bony casing of brain; blood flow to brain and related ICP are regulated by partial pressures of arterial carbon dioxide (PaCO$_2$) and oxygen (PaO$_2$), core body temperature, pH, and serum osmolality.

A. Pathophysiology: increased ICP; trauma, tumor, infection, anoxia, toxemia, and metabolic conditions
   1. Cerebral edema: elevated ICP; increase in brain volume caused by increase in brain water (see Nurse Alert, "Reducing Intracranial Pressure")

! N U R S E *A L E R T* !

Reducing Intracranial Pressure

To reduce intracranial pressure and promote jugular cerebral venous drainage, the nurse should:

- Elevate the head of the bed 30°–45°.
- Maintain the client's head and neck in midline alignment.
- Avoid rotating, flexing, or extending the client's neck.
- Avoid flexing the client's hips.
- Use a turn sheet when moving the client.
- Maintain a quiet, calm environment.

---

a) Vasogenic edema: most common type of fluid accumulation
   (1) Extracellular fluid volume increases with increase in plasma proteins.
   (2) Damaged blood vessels cause increased capillary permeability.
   (3) Causes include trauma, tumors, ischemia, infection, and abscess.
b) Cytogenic edema: intracellular edema; all brain components swell (e.g., neurons, glia, endothelial cells)
   (1) Sodium-potassium pump breaks down.
   (2) Potassium leaves cells; sodium and water enter.
   (3) Causes include both acute hypo-osmolality (e.g., hyponatremia) and hypoxia from trauma or cerebral hemorrhage.
c) Interstitial edema
   (1) Increase in extracellular fluid surrounding cells; buildup of fluid in ventricles of brain
   (2) Caused by obstruction and blockage of cerebrospinal fluid absorption (e.g., hydrocephalus, tumors, infection)
2. Central diabetes insipidus: inadequate production of ADH; polyuria and polydipsia; head trauma causes temporary brain swelling, preventing release of ADH; condition usually temporary
3. SIADH: excessive ADH production; head injury and subarachnoid hemorrhage among causes; resultant water retention exacerbates brain swelling; usually temporary

B. Nursing assessment
1. Assess for increased ICP; readings between 12 mm Hg and 19 mm Hg suggest elevated ICP, and readings above 20 mm Hg, definite ICP elevation.
2. Assess for changes in sensorium: headache, irritability, restlessness, confusion, and diplopia.
3. Assess for ophthalmic changes: unequal pupil size, decreased pupil response to light, and papilledema.
4. Assess for cardiac changes: bradycardia, increased systolic pressure, decreased diastolic pressure, widened pulse pressure, and atrial fibrillation.
5. Assess for changes in respiration: decreased or irregular respiration and pulmonary rales.
6. Assess for gastrointestinal changes: nausea and projectile vomiting.
7. Assess laboratory test values, with emphasis on $PaCO_2$, PaO_2, pH, and serum osmolality.
8. Reassess regularly for worsening conditions: discharge from nose and ears, apnea, and death.

C. Nursing diagnoses
1. Altered cerebral tissue perfusion related to cerebral edema secondary to head trauma or osmotic diuretic use
2. Hyponatremia related to SIADH or use of mannitol

3. High risk for ineffective breathing pattern related to cerebral edema and obstructed venous drainage
4. High risk for fluid and electrolyte imbalance related to fluid retention or osmotic diuresis or both
5. Altered sensorium related to cerebral edema
6. Altered urinary elimination, polyuria, related to central diabetes insipidus secondary to head trauma
7. Fluid volume excess related to SIADH secondary to head trauma

D. Nursing interventions
1. Monitor for changes in vital signs every 15–30 minutes.
2. Maintain patent airway and adequate ventilation.
3. Monitor level of consciousness; changes are often the first indication of elevated ICP.
4. Monitor sensory functions.
5. Monitor motor functions.
6. Monitor bowel sounds and functions; administer stool softeners as necessary.
7. Administer or restrict fluids, as ordered, carefully monitoring fluid status (e.g., IV fluids may cause fluid volume excess related to SIADH).
8. Monitor fluid intake, output, and urine specific gravity.
9. Administer corticosteroids (e.g., dexamethasone, methylprednisolone) or osmotic diuretics (e.g., mannitol, urea) or both on physician's orders; watch for cerebral rebleeding.
10. Monitor laboratory test values—including arterial blood gases—every 8 hours.
11. Instruct client on ways to avoid transient increases in ICP (see Client Teaching Checklist, "Preventing Transient Increases in Intracranial Pressure").

✔ CLIENT TEACHING CHECKLIST ✔

Preventing Transient Increases in Intracranial Pressure

To prevent transient increases in intracranial pressure, the nurse should instruct the client to:

✔ Avoid coughing or sneezing.
✔ Avoid bending or lifting.
✔ Exhale gently while changing position (holding the breath can increase intracranial pressure).
✔ Avoid straining for stools (stool softeners are generally prescribed to make straining unnecessary).

III. Shock: inadequate tissue oxygenation and insufficient waste excretion caused by circulatory collapse related to hypovolemia, failure of the pumping action of the heart, or failure of the peripheral resistance (determined by vascular tone and permeability)

See text pages

A. Pathophysiology
   1. Fluid and electrolyte effects
      a) Early shock: Fluid shifts from interstitial space to intravascular space to compensate for hypovolemia.
      b) Late shock: Fluid moves from intravascular space back into interstitial space.
      c) Sodium follows water.
   2. Cardiovascular effects: decreased arterial blood pressure compensated to normal or increased level in early shock by increased heart rate and vasoconstriction of blood vessels; falls in later shock as compensation fails
   3. Renal effects: decreased glomerular filtration, renal ischemia, and decreased urine output; kidney function compromised if systolic blood pressure falls below 60 mm Hg
   4. Types of shock
      a) Hypovolemic shock: low circulating blood volume; hemorrhage (external or internal), fluid loss (severe vomiting or diarrhea, dehydration), or fluid pooling (third-space shifts as seen with burns and intestinal obstruction; blood volume reduced by fluid shift)
      b) Cardiogenic shock: inadequate cardiac output; myocardial infarction, cardiac tamponade, cardiac failure, or pulmonary embolism
      c) Septic shock: increased capillary permeability; massive infection (usually gram-negative bacteria), peritonitis, or immunosuppressant therapy
      d) Neurogenic shock: loss of vascular tone and venous pooling of blood with vascular dilatation; extensive surgery, high spinal anesthesia, or severe emotional stress

B. Signs and symptoms (all types of shock unless noted)
   1. Respiration: increased rate and depth as compensation for decreasing pH
   2. Skin: pale, cold, and moist except in early septic shock, when skin is warm and flushed
   3. Pulse: fast and thready (tachycardia); early sign in all but neurogenic shock; due to release of epinephrine and norepinephrine
   4. Urinary output: decreased due to decreased renal blood flow
   5. Temperature: subnormal due to decreased circulation and metabolism except in septic shock, when temperature is elevated
   6. Muscular: weakness and fatigue due to buildup of lactic acid
   7. Sensorium: apprehension and restlessness progressing to disorientation and confusion; neurogenic shock excepted

8. Changes in blood pressure
   a) Pulse pressure (difference between systolic and diastolic pressures): diminished to less than 20 mm Hg
   b) Arterial blood pressure
      (1) Early shock: normal or elevated due to increased heart rate
      (2) Late shock: depressed due to inadequate circulatory volume
   c) Central venous pressure (CVP): decreased to less than 5 cm of water
   d) Pulmonary arterial pressure (PAP): decreased to less than 10 mm Hg in hypovolemic, septic, and neurogenic shock; increased to greater than 30 mm Hg in cardiogenic shock
   e) Pulmonary capillary wedge pressure (PCWP): decreased to less than 10 mm Hg in hypovolemic, neurogenic, and septic shock; increased to greater than 20 mm Hg in cardiogenic shock

C. Treatment and management
   1. Maintenance/restoration of adequate airway and respiration
   2. Body fluid maintenance to prevent tissue hypoxia: various fluids used (see Nurse Alert, "Blood and IV Calcium")
      a) Crystalloids: expand fluid in interstitial and intravascular spaces
         (1) Normal saline (0.9% sodium chloride [NaCl]): iso-osmolar; inexpensive; excess may cause hyperchloremia
         (2) Lactated Ringer's: buffers a pH decrease due to increased nonvolatile acid metabolites; large amounts cause metabolic alkalosis if liver function compromised
         (3) Normosol-R and Plasma-lyte R: contain additional electrolytes; expensive
      b) Colloids: substances whose size and molecular weight prohibit them from passing through the vascular membrane; increase intravascular fluid volume

! NURSE *ALERT* !

Blood and IV Calcium

When body fluid maintenance or replacement calls for blood transfusion in addition to IV fluid replacement, IV solutions that contain calcium (e.g., lactated Ringer's, Plasma-lyte R) should never be administered. Calcium forms a precipitate when it comes in contact with blood.

        (1) Examples: 5% or 25% albumin, 5% plasma protein fraction (natural products); hetastarch in 0.9% NaCl, dextran 40 or dextran 70 in either 0.9% NaCl or 5% dextrose in water (all synthetic products)

        (2) Advantages: less fluid needed to maintain volume; less chance of overhydration

        (3) Disadvantages: very expensive; use controversial; rapid administration can decrease blood pressure; dextran interferes with blood typing and cross matching

3. Specific measures for types of shock

   a) Hypovolemic shock: IV fluids (e.g., crystalloids, colloids, blood) to replace fluid volume and electrolytes; monitor blood gases; oxygen as needed; no vasopressors

   b) Cardiogenic shock: limited replacement of fluid volume; vasopressors if severe; drugs to prevent dysrhythmia and increase cardiac output; sedatives, diuretics, and oxygen

   c) Septic shock: culture for infectious agent; antibiotics with IV replacement therapy; steroids; vasopressors if no improvement

   d) Neurogenic shock: IV replacement therapy; sedatives for emotional shock; vasopressors if severe

D. Nursing process

  1. Nursing assessment

   a) Assess vital signs for symptoms of shock (e.g., tachycardia; rapid breathing; narrowed pulse pressure; cool, moist, pale skin).

   b) Obtain client's medical history, with emphasis on drugs that may precipitate shock or indicate a condition predisposing to shock (e.g., potassium-wasting diuretics, steroids, digitalis, antibiotics).

   c) Assess sensorium for signs of shock (e.g., restlessness, irritability).

   d) Obtain baseline values for laboratory tests.

  2. Nursing diagnoses

   a) Fluid volume deficit related to shock or trauma

   b) Fluid volume deficit related to massive infection

   c) Fluid volume excess related to excessive infusion of IV fluids

   d) Altered urinary elimination, oliguria, related to fluid volume deficit secondary to shock or trauma

   e) Altered tissue perfusion—renal, cerebral, or cardiopulmonary—related to decreased fluid volume secondary to shock or trauma

  3. Nursing interventions

   a) Monitor vital signs, and compare with baseline values.

   b) Monitor changes in skin color and turgor and in sensorium.

   c) Maintain accurate fluid intake and output records. Inform physician of urine output of less than 30 ml/hour.

   d) Monitor IV therapy, with special attention to changes in CVP and PCWP.

   e) Monitor changes in laboratory test results.

   f) Monitor changes in chest sounds for fluid volume overload.

See text pages
_____

IV. Burns

A. Pathophysiology

   1. Burn shock: fluid moves to burn site and into tissue spaces, where it is nonfunctional (third-space shift); hypovolemia; capillary permeability increased

   2. Decreased renal function: Hypovolemia results in oliguria aggravated by SIADH during first 48 hours; kidney damage may result.

   3. Hemolysis: destruction of red blood cells releases hemoglobin; excreted by kidney (red urine); kidney damage may result

B. Fluid and electrolyte imbalances

   1. Fluid accumulation phase: first 36–48 hours

     a) Intravascular fluid volume decreased as fluids shift into interstitial space

     b) Edema occurs at burn site; maximum rate of fluid accumulation by 6–8 hours postburn

     c) Sodium and water retained in response to aldosterone and ADH production; substantial decrease in urine output

     d) Serum osmolality and hematocrit increased due to loss of intravascular fluid

     e) Hyperkalemia due to potassium loss from cells coupled with reduced urinary excretion of potassium

     f) Hyponatremia due to rapid movement of sodium into edematous fluid; may last for weeks

     g) Metabolic acidosis due to nonvolatile acids released from injured cells and poor tissue perfusion

     h) Respiratory acidosis in inhalation injuries when pulmonary tissue is traumatized.

   2. Fluid remobilization phase: Diuresis begins about 48 hours postburn.

     a) Fluid moves back into intravascular space; edema at burn site decreases.

     b) Hypervolemia occurs if excessive IV fluids are administered.

     c) Hypokalemia occurs due to potassium-wasting diuretics, some antibiotics (e.g., sodium penicillin), and increased loss during diuresis.

     d) Hyponatremia may continue due to excessive free water intake (usually in children), use of aqueous silver nitrate dressings, loss of sodium during hydrotherapy, and loss of sodium during diuresis.

     e) Hypocalcemia may occur when calcium is sequestered in burned tissue.

     f) Hypomagnesemia may occur as a result of debridement and cleansing of burned tissue or from use of magnesium-wasting antibiotics (e.g., gentamicin).

g) Hypophosphatemia is related to excessive use of phosphate-binding antacids used to prevent gastric bleeding.

C. Signs and symptoms: severity of burns determined by depth, extent, cause of burn, client's age, and client's preexisting medical conditions
   1. Depth of burn
      a) Former classification system
         (1) First degree: pink, dry, slightly edematous; painful; only epidermis (outer layer of skin) damaged; of little clinical importance
         (2) Second degree: pink to deep red with blisters and capillary blanching; very painful; epidermis destroyed and dermis injured
         (3) Third degree: dry, without blisters, leathery, hard, white to charred; no sensation of pain; epidermis and dermis destroyed and subcutaneous tissue injured; new skin will not regenerate; no blanching
      b) Current classification system
         (1) Superficial: corresponds to first-degree burns
         (2) Partial thickness superficial: corresponds to severe first-degree and mild second-degree burns
         (3) Partial thickness deep: corresponds to moderate and severe second-degree burns; very painful
         (4) Full thickness: corresponds to third-degree burns
   2. Percentage of body surface area (BSA) burned: rule of nines; quick estimation of BSA based on multiples of nine; first-degree burn area

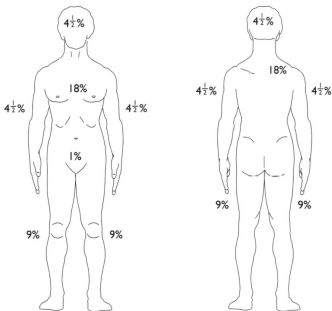

Figure 7–1
The Rule of Nines

not counted; useful only for adults with no preexisting medical
conditions; BSA estimates significantly inaccurate for children

- a) Head and neck total: 9%
    - (1) Anterior head and neck 4.5%
    - (2) Posterior head and neck 4.5%
- b) Upper extremities total: 18%
    - (1) Right arm anterior 4.5%, posterior 4.5%
    - (2) Left arm anterior 4.5%, posterior 4.5%
- c) Trunk and buttocks total: 36%
    - (1) Anterior 18%
    - (2) Posterior 18%
- d) Lower extremities total: 36%
    - (1) Right leg and thigh anterior 9%, posterior 9%
    - (2) Left leg and thigh anterior 9%, posterior 9%
- e) Genitals 1%

3. Classification of burn injury
    - a) Minor burn injury
        - (1) First degree
        - (2) Second degree covering BSA of less than 15% in adult
        - (3) Third degree covering BSA of less than 2%
    - b) Moderate burn injury
        - (1) Second degree covering BSA of 15%–25% in adult
        - (2) Second degree covering BSA of 10%–20% in child
        - (3) Third degree covering BSA of less than 10%
    - c) Major burn injury
        - (1) Second degree covering BSA of greater than 25% in adult
        - (2) Second degree covering BSA of greater than 20% in child
        - (3) Third degree covering BSA of greater than 10%
        - (4) Burns on hands, face, feet, or perineum
        - (5) Burns with inhalation injury
        - (6) Electrical burns
        - (7) Burns complicated by fractures or serious trauma
        - (8) All burns in children younger than 2, adults older than 60, and all others with preexisting medical conditions

4. Inhalation injuries: result from breathing in smoke or fumes; signs
include burns on face and neck, singed facial or nasal hair, any major
thermal burn from the waist up, and carbon in sputum
    - a) Carbon monoxide (CO): cherry-red skin; severe tachypnea or respiratory arrest
    - b) Smoke poisoning: signs appear within 24–48 hours of burn injury; increased mucous production, hoarseness, coughing,

labored or rapid breathing, rales, air hunger, and carbon in sputum

c) Circumferential third-degree burns of neck: edema causes pressure on trachea; hoarseness, dyspnea, stridor, restlessness, and air hunger

D. Treatment and management
  1. IV replacement therapy
    a) Necessary for moderate and critical burns: first- and second-degree burns covering more than 20% BSA or more than 10% BSA in children
    b) Adequacy of fluid replacement therapy monitored by hourly urine flow; desired rate in adult 30–50 ml/hour in early phase; may rise to 100 ml/hour in fluid mobilization phase
    c) Fluid replacement formulas
      (1) Many formulas are available, including Brook Army Hospital, Evans, Parkland, F. D. Moore, and Burnett Burn Center.
      (2) All seek to restore circulating blood volume.
      (3) All contain electrolytes and water.
      (4) Main difference is presence or absence of colloids (e.g., Parkland and Burnett Burn Center are colloid free).
  2. Fluid-accumulation-phase management goals
    a) Ensure adequate fluid volume replacement to maintain desirable urine output and prevent shock.
    b) Begin electrolyte replacement.
    c) Maintain sterility; begin antibiotic regimen.
    d) Prevent gastrointestinal complications.
    e) Maintain adequate oxygen and ventilation in inhalation injuries.
  3. Fluid-remobilization-phase management goals
    a) Prevent overhydration by significantly reducing or eliminating IV fluids.
    b) Provide diet for protein replacement.
    c) Maintain sterility.
  4. Convalescent-phase management goals
    a) Promote wound healing.
    b) Maintain sterility.
    c) Provide good nutrition and adequate electrolytes.
    d) Provide psychological support.

E. Nursing process
  1. Nursing assessment specific to burns
    a) Assess severity and extent of burn injury.
    b) Assess for burn shock, fluid volume deficit, and shock symptoms (see this chapter, section III,B).
    c) Assess for inhalation injuries (see section IV,C,4 of this chapter).

        d) Assess for gastrointestinal complications by looking for abdominal distension, absence of bowel sounds, nausea, vomiting, and blood in gastric secretions or stools.

        e) Assess for pain, whose severity varies with depth (inversely) and area of burn as well as individual pain threshold.

        f) Assess for disrupted skin integrity, which reduces antibacterial protection.

  2. Nursing diagnoses

        a) High risk for fluid volume deficit related to third-space shift secondary to major burns (fluid-accumulation phase)

        b) High risk for infection related to interrupted skin integrity

        c) High risk for fluid volume excess related to remobilization of sequestered fluids (fluid-remobilization phase)

        d) Altered urinary elimination, oliguria, related to hypovolemia secondary to shock, trauma, or burns

        e) Altered tissue perfusion related to hypovolemia secondary to shock, trauma, or burns

        f) High risk for ineffective breathing patterns related to burns of face, neck, and throat

        g) High risk for body image disturbance related to altered appearance from burns

        h) Pain

  3. Nursing interventions

        a) Initial interventions for burns

            (1) Stop further skin damage.

            (2) Keep airways open, and provide necessary assistance for continued breathing.

            (3) Establish replacement fluid therapy to improve circulation.

            (4) Institute aseptic procedures for burn areas; administer antibiotics.

            (5) Provide emotional support.

            (6) Monitor vital signs and laboratory test values.

            (7) Keep accurate fluid intake and output records.

        b) Additional interventions for inhalation injuries

            (1) Begin supplemental oxygen immediately.

            (2) Monitor swelling of neck and throat.

            (3) Supply high-humidity air.

            (4) Elevate head of bed.

            (5) Monitor for signs of smoke poisoning.

        c) Additional interventions for gastrointestinal complications

            (1) Monitor for signs of abdominal swelling.

            (2) Monitor for bowel sounds.

      (3) Monitor for signs of stomach bleeding.

      (4) Administer antacids or medication (e.g., cimetidine) to deter stomach bleeding.

      (5) Insert nasogastric tube on direction of physician.

  d) Additional interventions for pain

      (1) Administer analgesics.

      (2) Take safety precautions to avoid additional damage to burn areas.

  e) Additional interventions for disrupted skin integrity

      (1) Apply topical antibacterial agent to skin.

      (2) Vigorously maintain aseptic conditions and good wound-healing hygiene.

1. A client is receiving IV lactated Ringer's at 75 ml/hour to correct hypovolemia after an automobile accident. The client is in skeletal traction for a fractured femur. On the third posttrauma day, it will be especially important that the nurse monitor the client for:

   a. Hypocalcemia.
   b. Hypochloremia.
   c. Hypervolemia.
   d. Water intoxication.

2. A client is admitted to the emergency department after being struck by a car. The client is restless and disoriented, with a pulse (P) of 118 and blood pressure (BP) of 90/74. The most appropriate immediate treatment would be to administer:

   a. IV D_5W.
   b. IV normal saline.
   c. PO electrolyte solution.
   d. PO water.

3. An 87-year-old client sustained a head injury in a fall. The client is unconscious and ventilator dependent. Hyperventilation has been ordered to reduce a high intracranial pressure (ICP). Which of the following arterial blood gas (ABG) results should be reported to the physician immediately?

   a. HCO_3 = 20 mEq/L
   b. pH = 7.46
   c. $PaCO_2$ = 45 mm Hg
   d. PaO_2 = 75 mm Hg

4. Which of the following should the nursing care plan include for a client with high ICP?

   a. Maintaining client's head and neck in midline alignment
   b. Keeping head flat and legs elevated
   c. Client's performing range-of-motion exercises once per shift
   d. Encouraging coughing and deep breathing every 2 hours

5. A client has cerebral edema due to a skull fracture. IV mannitol is ordered, at a rate to be titrated to urine output. The client's urine output for the past hour was 20 ml. The nurse should:

   a. Increase the flow rate of the mannitol.
   b. Decrease the flow rate of the mannitol.
   c. Check the urine specific gravity.
   d. Discontinue the mannitol.

6. A client is hypovolemic. The client's BP is 86/40, central venous pressure (CVP) is 8 cm of water, and urine output has been 10–15 ml/hour. A fluid challenge is initiated. After administering 200 ml of normal saline over a period of 10 minutes, the nurse should evaluate CVP, BP, and:

   a. Lung sounds.
   b. Skin turgor.
   c. Temperature.
   d. Mental status.

7. A client has gram-negative septicemia and is at risk for septic shock. To detect early septic shock, the nurse should assess the client for:

   a. Cool, pale skin.
   b. Apprehension and restlessness.
   c. Elevated pulmonary capillary wedge pressure.
   d. Subnormal temperature.

8. A client is being treated for neurogenic shock with Levophed (levarterenol bitartrate). The flow rate of Levophed is titrated to maintain:

   a. Pulse rate below 120.
   b. Serum osmolality between 280 and 295 mOsm/kg.
   c. Urinary output of at least 30 ml/hour.
   d. Systolic BP of 80–90 mm Hg.

9. A client has second-degree burns over 30% of the body. Topical treatment with mafenide acetate (Sulfamylon) is immediately initiated. Fluid resuscitation with normal saline is in progress. No evidence of smoke inhalation is found. During the first 48 hours, for

which acid-base imbalance should the client be monitored?

a. Respiratory acidosis
b. Respiratory alkalosis
c. Metabolic acidosis
d. Metabolic alkalosis

10. By accidentally cutting an electrical line, a client sustains third-degree burns over 15% of the body. During the first 24 hours after the burn, which of the following nursing diagnoses would be appropriate for this client?

a. Decreased tissue perfusion related to edema of the burned tissues
b. Fluid volume excess related to postburn fluid shifts
c. Alteration in potassium balance (hypokalemia) related to renal excretion of excess potassium
d. Impaired gas exchange related to carbon monoxide inhalation

11. A client is receiving lactated Ringer's at 100 ml/hour to treat hypovolemia after a major burn. Which of the following assessment findings at 36 hours postburn indicates effective fluid therapy?

a. Systolic BP = 90 mm Hg
b. Apical pulse = 110
c. Capillary refill time = 7 seconds
d. Urine output = 50 ml/hour

12. A client sustained second- and third-degree burns of the legs. The client is currently receiving IV lactated Ringer's at 75 ml/hour. It is the third day postburn. The client is conscious and oriented. Which of the following fluid orders should the nurse anticipate at this time?

a. Switch to D_5W at 100 ml/hour.
b. Switch to 5% albumin at 50 ml/hour.
c. Discontinue IV fluids.
d. Continue present IV orders.

ANSWERS

1. **Correct answer is c.** On the second and third posttrauma days, fluid shifts back to the vascular space from the site of injury. Increased ADH and aldosterone after trauma promote fluid retention. If IV fluid administration is not decreased, hypervolemia is likely.

a. Hypercalcemia is more likely to occur during periods of immobilization.
b. Lactated Ringer's contains a concentration of chloride that is higher than normal serum levels. Hyperchloremia is more likely.
d. Water intoxication would occur if hypoosmolar fluid were given.

2. **Correct answer is b.** The client needs vascular volume expansion. Because normal saline is iso-osmolar, it would serve that purpose; it does not change serum osmolality. There would be no rapid fluid shifts between fluid compartments.

a. Dextrose would be rapidly metabolized, making the solution effectively hypoosmolar and lowering serum osmolality. Fluid would shift to the intracellular space.
c and d. Because surgery may be needed, the client should remain NPO.

3. **Correct answer is c.** The goal is to reduce the $PaCO_2$ (partial pressure of carbon dioxide in arterial blood) to 25–30 mm Hg to constrict cerebral vessels. A $PaCO_2$ on the high end of the normal range (35–45 mm Hg) indicates that the goal is not being achieved.

a. If the $PaCO_2$ is lowered, the kidneys compensate by excreting HCO_3 (bicarbonate). Such a below-normal value (normal range is 22–26 mEq/L) suggests that the treatment is working.
b. Before the kidneys have compensated, the pH would be slightly alkalotic, or above normal (7.35–7.45).
d. The elderly often have a PaO_2 (partial pressure of oxygen in arterial blood) below the normal adult range (80–100 mm Hg). A PaO_2 above 70 mm Hg is acceptable.

4. Correct answer is a. Rotation, flexion, and extension of the neck increase intracranial pressure. The head should be maintained in midline alignment.

b. The head of the bed should be elevated. Having the head flat and the legs elevated would increase ICP.
c. Range-of-motion exercises can increase ICP and are usually avoided while the ICP is elevated.
d. Coughing is contraindicated while the ICP is elevated, since it increases ICP.

5. Correct answer is d. Mannitol is usually titrated to maintain a urine output of 30–50 ml/hour. If renal function is not adequate to excrete the mannitol, hypervolemia and heart failure may develop. If urine output is below 30 ml/hour, mannitol should be discontinued and the physician notified.

a and b. Rate alteration is not appropriate. Mannitol must not be continued if renal function is inadequate.
c. Urine SG is assessed to evaluate hydration status. This will not help determine whether renal function is inadequate.

6. Correct answer is a. The development of crackles would indicate fluid overload. If crackles appear, the fluid challenge would be discontinued.

b. It may take 2–3 days for skin turgor to change; no effect would be detectable in 10 minutes.
c. Temperature change related to fluid volume status would not appear this quickly.
d. Mental status changes would indicate intracellular fluid excess. Normal saline expands vascular volume, so extracellular fluid status is monitored.

7. Correct answer is b. Apprehension and restlessness are early signs of developing shock.

a. Early in septic shock, the skin is warm and flushed due to vasodilation.

c. This occurs in cardiogenic shock. In other types of shock, pulmonary capillary wedge pressure drops.
d. In septic shock, the temperature remains elevated, due to fever.

8. Correct answer is d. Vasopressors are titrated based on systolic BP. To prevent cardiac dysrhythmias, the systolic BP should be maintained no higher than 90 mm Hg.

a. Vasopressors are catecholamines and increase pulse rate. Pulse is not used for titrating vasopressors.
b. Vasopressors do not alter fluid balance. Serum osmolality would not be an appropriate parameter for titrating vasopressor dosage.
c. Vasopressors constrict peripheral blood vessels, increasing BP. Urinary output may increase, but it is not the best parameter for titrating dosage.

9. Correct answer is c. Following a burn, nonvolatile, or fixed, acids released from injured tissues accumulate. Ineffective tissue perfusion causes hypoxia, which worsens acidosis. Sulfamylon's side effects include metabolic acidosis. If the kidneys cannot excrete chloride from normal saline, hyperchloremic acidosis may occur. This client has several risk factors for metabolic acidosis.

a. Because the client did not sustain smoke inhalation injuries, the risk for respiratory acidosis is not high.
b and d. Alkalosis is not a common acid-base imbalance in the early postburn period.

10. Correct answer is a. During the first 48 hours postburn, fluid shifts from the vessels to the interstitium at the burn site. Edema constricts the blood vessels in the area and would cause decreased tissue perfusion locally.

b. This nursing diagnosis is not appropriate until 48 hours postburn, when fluid shifts from the interstitium back to the vessels.

c. In the early postburn period, especially after electrical burns, potassium is released from damaged tissues, causing hyperkalemia. Later, the kidneys excrete excess potassium, and hypokalemia may develop.
d. Carbon monoxide inhalation is related to smoke exposure. In the case of an electrical burn, smoke inhalation is not a factor.

11. **Correct answer is d.** The most useful parameter for monitoring effectiveness of fluid therapy after a burn is urine output. Urine output between 30 and 50 ml/hour indicates effective therapy.

    a. Systolic BP should remain close to normal if fluid replacement is adequate. A systolic BP less than 100 mm Hg should be reported to the physician.
    b. Tachycardia is expected in the first few hours postburn. At 36 hours, tachycardia most likely indicates hypovolemia.
    c. Normal capillary refill time is less than 3 seconds. Prolonged capillary refill time indicates hypovolemia or impaired tissue perfusion.

12. **Correct answer is c.** At about 48 hours postburn, the fluid remobilization phase begins. As edema fluid returns to circulation, there is a risk of circulatory overload. If oral intake is possible, IV fluids will probably be discontinued.

    a. During the fluid remobilization phase, a reduction of IV rate is indicated. D_5W is appropriate for part of the fluid replacement in the first 24 hours. It is not indicated on the third day postburn.
    b. Colloids may be used during the first 48 hours to help retain fluid in the vascular space. Colloids would not be appropriate in the fluid remobilization phase.
    d. The rate of fluid administration should be reduced in the fluid remobilization phase if IV fluids are still needed. This client is conscious, so oral intake should be sufficient.

8

Gastrointestinal and Related Problems

NURSING HIGHLIGHTS

1. The electrolyte and metabolic imbalances that occur with GI problems vary with the type of fluid lost; the composition and pH of gastric fluids are significantly different from the composition and pH of intestinal fluids.
2. The nurse can decrease the chance of fluid and electrolyte complications after major GI surgery by making sure the client is properly rehydrated and maintained before the operation.
3. Clients with cirrhosis must be monitored closely for decreasing responsiveness to diuretics and increasing ascites and edema.
4. Pain is a significant factor affecting respiration depth and hence acid-base metabolism in both GI surgery and pancreatitis.

constipation—decreased frequency of bowel movements accompanied by prolonged or difficult evacuation of stools; caused by medications, psychologic or mechanical disorders, or metabolic disorders such as dehydration

fistula—abnormal connection between intestinal tract and skin (external fistula) or intestinal tract and a body cavity (internal fistula)

paracentesis—surgical puncture of a body cavity to remove accumulated fluid

peristalsis—waves of alternating circular contractions through a muscular tube that move the contents forward

ENHANCED OUTLINE

I. Gastrointestinal (GI) problems: large volumes of fluid pass into the GI tract and are reabsorbed during normal digestion; excess fluid loss most common abnormality

See text pages

A. Vomiting and gastric suction
    1. Fluid and electrolyte considerations
        a) pH of GI fluids
            (1) Saliva 6.0–7.0
            (2) Gastric juice 1.0–3.5
            (3) Pancreatic juice 8.0–8.3
            (4) Bile 5.0–6.0
            (5) Small intestine 7.5–8.0
            (6) Large intestine 7.5–8.0
        b) Major electrolytes: hydrogen, chloride, potassium, and sodium
    2. Fluid and electrolyte disturbances
        a) Fluid volume deficit (FVD): due to severe vomiting or gastric suction
        b) Metabolic alkalosis: due to loss of chloride in gastric juice, with compensatory increase in bicarbonate; kidneys fail to excrete bicarbonate excess; side effect is decrease in ionized calcium with increased neuromuscular excitability
        c) Hypokalemia: due to loss of high-potassium gastric fluid
        d) Sodium imbalances
            (1) Hyponatremia usually related to excessive free water intake (e.g., IV 5% dextrose in water) in hospitalized clients losing gastric fluid to gastric suction or excessive vomiting
            (2) Hypernatremia related to gastric fluid loss coupled with free water losses (e.g., hyperventilation, fever)
        e) Hypomagnesemia: due to prolonged gastric suction
    3. Management for gastric fluid loss by vomiting
        a) Promote frequent intake of small amounts of fluids containing electrolytes.

   b) Report vomiting so that physician can prescribe antinausea medication.

   c) Remove environmental stimuli that encourage vomiting (e.g., strong odors).

   d) Encourage bed rest, because rapid movements stimulate vomiting.

   e) Keep accurate fluid intake and output records.

   f) Monitor daily for fluid-related weight changes.

  4. Management for gastric fluid loss by gastric suction

   a) Irrigate suction tube with isotonic fluids to prevent electrolyte washout.

   b) Limit the amount of water or ice taken by mouth.

   c) Keep accurate record of fluid loss by suction.

   d) Monitor daily for fluid-related weight changes.

 B. Diarrhea: Causes include viral and bacterial infections, parasites, and drugs.

  1. Types of diarrhea

   a) Osmotic: High osmolality of bowel contents draws water into bowel; causes include general malabsorption as well as ingestion of poorly absorbed substances (e.g., lactulose, mannitol).

   b) Secretory: abnormal secretion of water and electrolytes into bowel; causes include infectious agents (e.g., *Escherichia coli*), severe hypoalbuminemia, and intestinal obstruction

   c) Structural: Causes include inflammatory bowel disease and sprue.

   d) Primary motility disorders: adynamic ileus and paralytic ileus

  2. Fluid and electrolyte imbalances

   a) FVD: Severe diarrhea can cause fluid and electrolyte loss of 2–10 liters/day.

   b) Metabolic acidosis: common, especially in infants and children; due to loss of alkaline intestinal fluid

   c) Hypokalemia: due to loss of potassium-rich intestinal fluid

   d) Hypomagnesemia: due to loss of magnesium-rich intestinal fluid

   e) Sodium imbalances: Either hyponatremia or hypernatremia may result depending on relative losses of water and sodium.

  3. Management of diarrhea

   a) Offer small amounts of electrolyte-containing fluids if bowel does not need to rest.

   b) Keep accurate fluid intake and output records.

   c) Monitor fluid status; parenteral fluids may be prescribed if bowel needs prolonged rest.

   d) Monitor body weight for fluid-related weight changes.

e) Provide soft foods first when oral foods are permitted; BRAT diet (bananas, rice, applesauce, toast) is appropriate.

C. Bowel preparation for diagnostic tests and surgery: elderly at risk for fluid and electrolyte imbalances (see Chapter 6, section II,B,6)
   1. Colon cleansing by clear liquid diet: 1–3 days plus laxatives and enemas; disadvantages include weakness due to lengthy period needed to cleanse bowel as well as electrolyte imbalances caused by laxatives and enemas (see this chapter, section I,D)
   2. Colon cleansing by polyethylene glycol (PEG) solution: 1.5 liters/hour (up to 4 liters) until bowel effluent is clear
      a) Advantages: even large volumes have little effect on fluid and electrolyte balance; shorter period needed to cleanse bowel
      b) Disadvantages: may cause nausea, abdominal fullness, or bloating; fluid and electrolyte imbalances possible
   3. Enemas for bowel cleansing (see this chapter, section I,D,2, for fluid and electrolyte considerations in enema use)

D. Laxatives and enemas for constipation: preferred treatment is through diet and nonpharmacologic interventions (see Nurse Alert, "Avoiding Laxative and Enema Dependence")
   1. Laxatives: Chronic use can lead to fluid and electrolyte imbalances.
      a) Isotonic dehydration: Both water and sodium are lost.
      b) Hypermagnesemia: likely with impaired renal function or poor bowel motility when laxative contains magnesium salts (e.g., magnesium citrate, milk of magnesia)
      c) Hyperphosphatemia: likely with impaired renal function when laxative contains sodium phosphate
   2. Enemas
      a) Multiple tap water enemas may produce hyponatremia due to absorption of plain water; especially common in children

---

! **NURSE ALERT** !

Avoiding Laxative and Enema Dependence

To help clients achieve normal, comfortable bowel movements without pharmacologic intervention, the nurse should:

- Encourage regular, moderate physical activity such as walking.
- Encourage clients to drink a glass of warm liquid in the morning to stimulate the evacuation response.
- Promote regular fluid intake to soften stools.
- Encourage clients to eat a diet high in fiber (e.g., whole-grain cereals, fruits, vegetables).
- Encourage clients to establish a regular time for bowel elimination; usually just after breakfast is most effective.

      b) Hypertonic sodium phosphate enemas (e.g., Fleet) may produce hyperphosphatemia, hypocalcemia, and hypernatremia in clients who have difficulty eliminating enema solution; use cautiously in clients with heart disease, renal impairment, or preexisting electrolyte imbalances and in clients using diuretics or calcium channel blockers.

      c) Adult-size enemas ought never to be used for infants or children; may cause hyperphosphatemia, hypocalcemia, acidosis, or shock

E. Fistulas: result from trauma (e.g., surgery) or as a complication of disease (e.g., pancreatitis, inflammatory bowel syndrome)
   1. Metabolic acidosis: high loss of bicarbonate in intestinal fluids
   2. Metabolic alkalosis: high loss of hydrogen ions in gastric fluid
   3. Fluid and electrolyte imbalances: FVD and hyponatremia

F. Bulimia nervosa: eating disorder in which eating binges alternate with self-induced vomiting; abuse of laxatives, diuretics, and diet pills; fasting
   1. Most common in women in their late teens and early 20s
   2. Fluid and electrolyte imbalances: FVD, hypochloremic metabolic alkalosis, hypokalemia, hyponatremia, and metabolic acidosis

G. Intestinal obstruction: complete or partial
   1. Mechanical obstruction: Adhesions, hernia, tumor, or diverticula block normal passage of intestinal contents.
      a) Simple blockage: Vascular supply remains intact.
      b) Strangulated blockage: Vascular supply is inhibited.
      c) Gas and fluid collection behind obstruction: Fluid accumulates faster than it is absorbed.
        (1) Third-space shift occurs (6 liters or more of fluid may accumulate).
        (2) Reduction of intravascular fluid volume results in hypovolemic shock.
   2. Functional obstruction (paralytic ileus or adynamic ileus): ineffective or nonproductive peristalsis; motor activity slowed but not totally absent
      a) Fluid accumulation due to decreased absorption
      b) Electrolyte imbalances
        (1) Hyponatremia: Client becomes thirsty and drinks water, diluting serum sodium.
        (2) Metabolic alkalosis: Client vomits gastric juice due to pyloric or high intestinal (jejunal) obstruction.
        (3) Metabolic acidosis: Client vomits intestinal juice due to low intestinal obstruction.

II. GI surgery: interrupts ingestion, absorption, and transportation of fluids and nutrients

See text pages

_____

A. Fluid and electrolyte imbalances
1. Preoperative conditions affecting fluid and electrolyte balance
    a) Preexisting imbalances due to vomiting, diarrhea, or intestinal obstruction
    b) Preoperative preparation (e.g., bowel cleansing, gastric or intestinal intubation)
2. Postoperative conditions affecting fluid and electrolyte balance
    a) Third-space shifts
    b) Restrictions on fluid intake
    c) Drainage through GI tubes
    d) Interrupted or sluggish peristalsis or both
    e) Disturbed breathing patterns due to narcotics or pain
3. Common imbalances
    a) Hypovolemia related to intravascular fluid shift to third space
    b) Fluid volume excess (FVE): sodium and water retained; usually iatrogenic if intravascular
    c) Hypokalemia: excessive urinary and GI potassium losses
    d) Metabolic acidosis: high loss of intestinal fluid
    e) Metabolic alkalosis: high loss of gastric juice

B. Management
1. Preoperative
    a) Use fluid and electrolyte therapy to stabilize client before surgery.
    b) Monitor renal output.
    c) Prepare client for operation by means of bowel cleansing regimen or gastric or intestinal intubation as needed.
2. Postoperative
    a) Maintain fluid and electrolyte therapy; adjust as indicated by laboratory tests.
    b) Monitor fluid intake (parenteral) and output.
    c) Maintain gastric drainage tube; monitor fluid volume and composition; limit irrigation with plain water.
    d) Maintain client NPO or with limited water by mouth only to alleviate discomfort.
    e) Provide antibiotics as ordered by physician.
    f) Encourage client to breathe deeply to prevent respiratory acidosis.

C. Nursing process
1. Nursing assessment
    a) Assess client's health status with respect to preexisting fluid and electrolyte imbalances; preexisting cardiac, renal, pulmonary, or endocrine disease; and medications affecting fluid and electrolyte balance.
    b) Assess vital signs, with emphasis on blood pressure, pulse rate, rhythm, and volume to determine baseline values.

      c) Assess laboratory test values.

      d) Assess fluid volume status, noting intake and output, including losses from diaphoresis and drainage from dressings.

      e) Assess patency of GI tubes.

2. Nursing diagnoses

      a) Fluid volume deficit related to excessive loss of GI fluid, decreased fluid intake and/or third-space fluid volume shift

      b) High risk for ineffective airway clearance related to pain, narcotic administration, ineffective breathing patterns, and/or pulmonary secretions

      c) Pain related to trauma of GI surgery

      d) Pain related to decreased bowel motility and absence of bowel sounds

3. Nursing interventions

      a) Monitor fluid and electrolyte status; provide parenteral fluids as ordered by physician.

      b) Monitor vital signs, with special attention to changes in cardiac function indicating fluid volume imbalances.

      c) Elevate the head of the bed, and encourage client to breathe deeply and change positions frequently.

      d) Observe for signs of respiratory distress; suction to keep airways clear.

      e) Treat cause of pain with medication or diversion or both; must manage well to promote deep breathing, coughing, and the ambulation needed to prevent pulmonary complications

---

See text pages

III. Cirrhosis of the liver: Liver becomes fibrous, compressing blood, lymph, and biliary channels and reducing the liver's capacity to function.

A. Pathophysiology and etiology

1. Causes of cirrhosis: chemicals and drugs toxic to the liver; alcoholism, especially with malnutrition; viral hepatitis; obstruction of bile flow

2. Ascites formation: Serous fluid accumulates in peritoneal cavity.

      a) Early cirrhosis: Baroreceptor reflex increases sodium and water retention, expanding plasma volume.

      b) Advanced cirrhosis: Fluid overflow spills into peritoneal cavity.

3. Physiologic basis of cirrhosis

      a) Portal vein pressure increases (portal obstruction hypertension) because of impeded flow through fibrous liver.

      b) Total extracellular fluid volume remains normal or increases, but arterial volume reaching kidneys decreases.

      c) Capillary permeability increases.

      d) Increased aldosterone production increases sodium and water retention.

      e) Serum albumin and serum protein decrease as protein-synthesizing capacity of liver declines.

      f) Plasma oncotic pressure decreases due to hypoalbuminemia and hypoproteinemia, allowing fluid to move into peritoneal space.

      g) Pitting edema occurs secondary to increased venous pressure and hypoproteinemia.

B. Signs and symptoms

  1. GI: bleeding esophageal varices (enlarged blood vessels), anorexia, vomiting, diarrhea, abdominal pain, ascites, constipation, and weight loss (all exacerbated by malnutrition)

  2. Renal

    a) Oliguria related to decreased glomerular filtration and increased water retention

    b) Hepatorenal syndrome (HRS): end-stage hepatic failure; serum creatinine greater than 1.5 mg/dl; blood urea nitrogen greater than 25 mg/dl; usually fatal

  3. Cardiovascular: dysrhythmia due to abnormal potassium levels; changes related to circulating blood volume decrease

  4. Neurologic

    a) Portal systemic encephalopathy (PSE)

      (1) Confusion and disturbed consciousness: accumulation of toxins (e.g., ammonia) normally destroyed by the liver

      (2) Sleep disorders (mild) to seizures and coma (severe)

      (3) Contributing factors: FVD due to excess use of diuretics, high dietary protein, GI bleeding (digestion yields ammonia), infection, constipation, progressive liver failure, and hypokalemia with metabolic alkalosis

    b) Other neurologic changes: paresthesia, sensory disturbances, peripheral nerve degeneration, and palsy of the sixth cranial nerve

  5. Respiratory: lung capacity decreased due to upward pressure from ascites, or ascites fluid leaking into pleural (lung) cavity, or both; pulmonary hypertension; and hyperventilation with respiratory alkalosis due to increased ammonia levels

  6. Skin: jaundice (total serum bilirubin elevated to greater than 3.0 mg/dl), mottled red spots on palms (palmar erythema), vascular spiders (bluish-red dilated superficial blood vessels), and pitting edema

  7. Blood: anemia, increased rate of red blood cell destruction, and increased clotting time resulting in prolonged bleeding

  8. Fluid and electrolyte

    a) Increased extracellular fluid volume accompanied by decreased effective arterial volume

    b) Hyponatremia: More water is retained than sodium.

    c) Hypokalemia: potassium loss through vomiting or diarrhea; loss through potassium-wasting diuretics; decreased dietary intake

        d) Hyperkalemia: excess use of potassium-sparing diuretics coupled with renal impairment

        e) Hypomagnesemia: magnesium loss through vomiting or diarrhea; decreased dietary intake

        f) Hypocalcemia: possibly due to inadequate storage of vitamin D by liver

        g) Increased serum ammonia: Liver fails to convert ammonia to urea for excretion.

C. Treatment and management: control FVE (e.g., ascites, edema)

   1. Sodium restriction: 500–1000 mg/day; constitutes sufficient treatment, in conjunction with bed rest, for some clients with cirrhosis

   2. Fluid restriction: 1000–1500 ml/day

   3. Diuretic use

        a) Excess use may result in hypovolemia.

        b) Spironolactone (aldosterone antagonist) may be alternated with potassium-wasting diuretics (e.g., furosemide, bumetanide).

   4. Paracentesis: may be needed for ascites causing respiratory distress or intra-abdominal pressure (clients often become refractory to diuretics); excessive fluid removal can cause circulatory collapse

   5. Peritoneal venous shunt (e.g., LeVeen shunt, Denver shunt): Shunt redirects ascitic fluid back into venous system.

D. Nursing process

   1. Nursing assessment specific to cirrhotic clients

        a) Assess urine output; notify physician if output is less than 30 ml/hour.

        b) Assess for pitting edema in lower extremities.

        c) Determine baseline weight.

        d) Measure abdominal girth; mark tape placement, at midline and both sides, to ensure consistency for serial measurements.

        e) Assess skin for vascular spiders, palmar erythema, and jaundice.

        f) Assess neurologic status.

   2. Nursing diagnoses

        a) Fluid volume excess with decreased effective arterial volume related to changes in liver

        b) Risk for impaired gas exchange related to reduced lung expansion secondary to pressure from ascites

        c) Altered thought processes related to accumulation of toxins (e.g., ammonia)

        d) Altered thought processes related to hyponatremia

        e) Altered nutrition, less than body requirements, related to alcoholism and inadequate intake

        f) Risk for injury related to changes in neurologic status

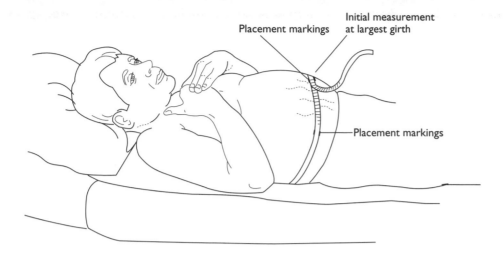

Figure 8–1
Measuring Abdominal Girth

3. Nursing interventions specific to cirrhotic clients
    a) Monitor fluid balance by using daily changes in weight and abdominal girth as well as standard intake and output records.
    b) Monitor for changes in vital signs and laboratory test values.
    c) Monitor for signs of portal systemic encephalopathy, especially if client has GI bleeding.
    d) Take safety precautions if client has changes in neurologic status.

IV. Pancreatitis: inflammation of the pancreas

See text pages
_____

A. Pathophysiology and etiology
    1. Damage to pancreas releases enzymes causing edema, ischemia, and necrosis as enzymes digest pancreatic and surrounding tissues.
    2. Alcoholism is leading cause of pancreatitis.
    3. 60% of nonalcoholic clients with pancreatitis have gallstones; physiologic connection is unclear.
    4. Other causes may include trauma, surgery, drugs, and Coxsackie virus

B. Fluid and electrolyte imbalances
    1. Edema in area of pancreas: Fluid shifts from vascular space as result of peritoneal burn caused by release of pancreatic enzymes.
    2. Hypovolemia: due to third-space shift; plasma volume may decrease 30%–40% in 6 hours
    3. Hypocalcemia and hypomagnesemia: may be due to precipitation of calcium and magnesium ions in damaged pancreatic tissue and/or related to hypoalbuminemia

    4. Respiratory alkalosis: hyperventilation stimulated by pain

    5. Metabolic alkalosis: severe vomiting and gastric suction

    6. Metabolic acidosis: renal failure due to severe hypovolemia

C. Treatment and management

    1. Maintain adequate circulating blood volume by IV fluid replacement.

    2. Administer parenteral electrolytes including calcium and magnesium.

    3. Manage severe pain with medication and use of nasogastric tube.

    4. Control nausea and vomiting with nasogastric suction.

    5. Provide respiratory support as needed.

    6. Provide nutrition through total parenteral nutrition (TPN) or enteral feeding tube to jejunum (nasojejunal tube) until pancreas has rested.

D. Nursing process

    1. Nursing assessment

       a) Assess vital signs, fluid intake and output, and laboratory test values.

       b) Assess for signs of hypovolemia.

       c) Assess for signs of hemorrhagic shock.

       d) Assess for signs of respiratory distress.

       e) Assess client's sensorium.

       f) Assess for infection (e.g., pancreatic abscess).

    2. Nursing diagnoses

       a) Fluid volume deficit related to third-space shift and vomiting or gastric suction

       b) Ineffective breathing pattern related to pain and fluid in pleural cavity

       c) Altered nutrition, less than body requirements, related to prolonged NPO period

       d) Pain related to pancreatic disease

    3. Nursing interventions specific to pancreatitis

       a) Collaborate with physician in administering fluid and electrolyte replacement therapy.

       b) Monitor vital signs, laboratory test values, and fluid intake and output.

       c) Maintain patency of nasogastric suction tube.

       d) Provide nutrition support (TPN, jejunal feeding), as ordered.

       e) Implement measures to relieve pain.

       f) Minimize respiratory complications by turning client regularly, encouraging deep breathing, and keeping airways open.

       g) Provide rest periods and a quiet, calm environment.

1. A client has gastroenteritis. The client has been vomiting for 2 days and is unable to take oral fluids. IV half-strength saline is ordered. The nurse should consult the physician for orders to supplement which electrolyte?

   a. Sodium
   b. Phosphorus
   c. Calcium
   d. Potassium

2. A client has Crohn's disease with chronic diarrhea. Which of the following nursing diagnoses is most likely to be appropriate for this client?

   a. Alteration in acid-base balance (metabolic acidosis) related to loss of intestinal fluids
   b. Alteration in potassium balance (hyperkalemia) related to renal potassium retention with bicarbonate
   c. Alteration in acid-base balance (metabolic alkalosis) related to excessive chloride loss in diarrhea
   d. Alteration in calcium balance (hypercalcemia) related to loss of phosphorus in diarrhea

3. An 80-year-old client is to take GoLytely, a polyethylene glycol (PEG) solution—ordered before a colonoscopy. The nurse should instruct the client to:

   a. Take GoLytely with a high-protein meal.
   b. Follow a clear liquid diet for 24 hours before taking GoLytely.
   c. Chill GoLytely in the refrigerator before taking it.
   d. Take nothing by mouth after taking GoLytely.

4. A client is at risk for fluid volume deficit and electrolyte imbalances due to frequent laxative use. To reduce dependence on laxatives the nurse should teach this client to:

   a. Include an iced beverage with breakfast.
   b. Plan daily exercise such as walking.
   c. Avoid gas-forming foods such as cabbage, broccoli, and beans.
   d. Limit intake of water and to drink juices instead.

5. A client had surgical treatment for a gunshot wound. A fistula has developed between the duodenum and the abdominal wall. The nurse should monitor this client for:

   a. Postural hypotension.
   b. Slow, shallow respirations.
   c. Flaccid leg muscles.
   d. Peripheral edema.

6. A client is admitted to the psychiatric unit for treatment of bulimia nervosa. The client has used laxatives and diuretics for weight loss. On the third day in the hospital, the client complains of a bloated feeling and has peripheral edema. The nurse should advise this client to:

   a. Limit fluid intake.
   b. Avoid adding salt to food.
   c. Eat more complex carbohydrates.
   d. Reduce protein intake.

7. A client returns from surgery with a nasogastric (NG) tube to continuous suction after a bowel resection. The physician's orders include "ice chips sparingly to relieve dry mouth." Which of the following should the nurse do?

   a. Offer the client a 1-oz cup of ice chips each hour.
   b. Provide a pitcher of ice chips and tell the client to use them sparingly.
   c. Irrigate the NG tube with normal saline each time the client takes ice chips.
   d. Clamp the NG tube for 15 minutes each time the client takes ice chips.

8. A 70-year-old client had a cholecystectomy today. To minimize the client's risk for respiratory acidosis, the nursing care plan should include:
   a. Positioning a pillow to splint the client's incision at all times.
   b. Coaching the client to take deep breaths—without coughing—every hour.
   c. Elevating the head of the bed 45°.
   d. Limiting fluid intake to an amount equal to the client's urine output.

9. A client has ascites secondary to cirrhosis. Which of the following foods should the nurse advise this client to avoid?
   a. Fresh grapefruit sections
   b. All-beef hot dogs
   c. Cooked frozen spinach
   d. Horseradish for seasoning

10. A client has a paracentesis, during which 4 liters of ascitic fluid are removed. Immediately after the paracentesis, the nurse must monitor the client closely for:
    a. Deteriorating mental status.
    b. Respiratory distress.
    c. Circulatory collapse.
    d. Disseminated intravascular coagulation.

11. A client has portal systemic encephalopathy secondary to cirrhosis. Lactulose is prescribed. If the dosage is appropriate, which of the following outcomes will the nurse note?
    a. A liquid stool after each dose
    b. Between 4 and 6 watery stools daily
    c. A formed stool daily
    d. Either 2 or 3 soft stools daily

12. Which of the following nursing diagnoses is most appropriate for a client with acute pancreatitis on admission?
    a. Alteration in calcium balance (hypercalcemia) related to insufficient parathyroid hormone
    b. Alteration in magnesium balance (hypermagnesemia) related to elevated blood sugar

    c. Fluid volume excess: peripheral edema related to decreased serum albumin
    d. Fluid volume deficit: hypovolemia related to third-space shifts in response to inflammation

ANSWERS

1. **Correct answer is d.** Gastric fluids lost in vomiting are rich in potassium and magnesium. Both may need to be supplemented in prolonged vomiting.

   a. Gastric fluid is either iso-osmolar or hypo-osmolar, so serum sodium usually remains normal.
   b and **c.** Gastric fluids are not high in phosphorus or calcium.

2. **Correct answer is a.** Losses of alkaline intestinal fluid produce metabolic acidosis.

   b. Hypokalemia is likely because intestinal fluids are high in potassium. Sodium, not potassium, is resorbed with bicarbonate.
   c. Chloride is retained as bicarbonate is lost, contributing to metabolic acidosis.
   d. Calcium levels do increase as phosphorus is lost, but diarrhea does not cause loss of large amounts of phosphorus.

3. **Correct answer is c.** Chilling the solution improves its palatability.

   a. The manufacturers of PEG solutions recommend avoiding solid food for 3–4 hours before taking those solutions.
   b. One advantage of PEG solutions is that the traditional 1–3 days of clear liquid diet are not required.
   d. Clear liquids are usually permitted after taking PEG solutions. The elderly are at risk for hypovolemia when fluids are restricted.

4. **Correct answer is b.** Exercise enhances peristalsis. Walking is especially effective to prevent constipation, because it strengthens abdominal muscles.

a. Hot beverages stimulate peristalsis. Iced beverages have no benefit.

c. All of these are sources of fiber, which helps prevent constipation. They do not need to be avoided unless flatulence is a problem.

d. Avoiding water is likely to decrease total fluid intake. Fluids help soften the stool, preventing constipation.

5. **Correct answer is a.** A duodenal fistula can drain as much as 4 liters of fluid daily. Postural hypotension is an early sign of fluid volume deficit.

   b. Hypochloremia and metabolic alkalosis cause slow, shallow respirations. Because intestinal fluid does not contain large amounts of chloride, this is unlikely.

   c. This is a sign of hyperkalemia. Because large amounts of potassium are lost in intestinal fluid, the client is at risk for hypokalemia.

   d. Peripheral edema occurs with fluid volume excess.

6. **Correct answer is b.** Reflex fluid retention often occurs when laxative or diuretic abuse is abruptly discontinued. Salt restriction may help reduce it.

   a. Fluids should not be limited. Laxative and diuretic abuse cause fluid volume deficits. Fluid needs to be replaced.

   c. Complex carbohydrates do not alter fluid balance.

   d. This client's efforts at weight control may have caused protein depletion. Low albumin levels contribute to edema. Increased protein would help replace the deficient albumin.

7. **Correct answer is a.** As water from the ice chips is suctioned from the stomach, it carries electrolytes with it. To prevent electrolyte deficits, the amount of ice chips should be limited.

   b. The nurse should provide only small amounts of ice chips. The term *sparingly* is vague and may be interpreted various ways. The client's judgment is impaired by effects of anesthesia and pain medication.

c. Irrigation solution is quickly removed, so it is not absorbed to replace electrolytes.

d. Until peristalsis returns, fluids taken orally are not absorbed, but remain in the stomach until they are suctioned out. Longer retention in the stomach would permit more electrolyte depletion.

8. **Correct answer is c.** Shallow breathing due to age-related changes and the high incision cause carbon dioxide (CO_2) retention and respiratory acidosis. Elevating the head of the bed promotes lung expansion and CO_2 excretion.

   a. The incision should be splinted to reduce pain with deep breathing and coughing. Constant splinting would restrict lung expansion, causing CO_2 retention.

   b. Coughing is important to reduce retention of secretions that would further impair CO_2 excretion.

   d. Fluid intake needs to be at least 500 ml/day more than output to replace surgical losses. Increased fluids help to mobilize respiratory secretions.

9. **Correct answer is b.** Processed meats, such as hot dogs, contain large amounts of sodium. Patients with ascites need to be on sodium-restricted diets.

   a. Citrus fruits are high in potassium. High aldosterone levels in cirrhosis produce hypokalemia. High-potassium foods should be encouraged unless renal failure is present.

   c. Frozen vegetables are not high in sodium. Canned vegetables are.

   d. Horseradish is one of the few low-sodium seasonings available. Its use may help make low-sodium foods palatable.

10. **Correct answer is c.** When paracentesis removes large volumes of fluid, ascites may rapidly reaccumulate, depleting vascular volume severely. Circulatory collapse is possible.

    a. This would occur with elevated blood ammonia or dilutional hyponatremia. Neither is a complication of paracentesis.

b. Respiratory distress is more likely before the paracentesis, when ascites would limit lung expansion.

d. Disseminated intravascular coagulation is a complication of peritoneovenous shunts, which may introduce foreign matter from ascitic fluid into the bloodstream.

11. **Correct answer is d.** Lactulose is given to reduce intestinal pH so less ammonia is absorbed. Its osmotic effect also increases the water content of stools. At the appropriate dose, 2 or 3 soft stools daily are expected.

a and **b.** These outcomes reflect excessive dosage. Diarrhea depletes electrolytes and fluid and must be avoided.

c. This would reflect an appropriate laxative dose, but a higher dose is needed to reduce ammonia absorption.

12. **Correct answer is d.** Autodigestion releases pancreatic enzymes that induce an inflammatory response in the pancreas and peritoneum. As much as 10 liters of fluid may be sequestered in these areas of inflammation.

a. Hypocalcemia is seen with pancreatitis. Deficient parathyroid hormone, albumin, and magnesium as well as excess calcitonin and glucagon all may contribute to it.

b. Hypomagnesemia develops as magnesium precipitates in inflamed tissues. Vomiting, gastric suction, and diarrhea also cause magnesium loss.

c. Serum albumin levels drop in pancreatitis. However, because the patient is hypovolemic, peripheral edema does not develop.

9

Cardiopulmonary Problems

NURSING HIGHLIGHTS

1. Left-sided heart failure symptoms are generally those of fluid volume overload; right-sided heart failure symptoms have to do with increased pulmonary pressure; left-sided and right-sided failure can occur simultaneously.
2. Congestive heart failure can be either chronic or acute.
3. The nurse should be alert for signs of compensation in early congestive heart failure.
4. Management of congestive heart failure is aimed at reducing the workload of the heart.
5. Management of chronic obstructive pulmonary disease is aimed at increasing gas exchange in the lungs.

GLOSSARY

diastole—the dilation of the heart chambers during which they fill with blood
Fowler's position—an inclined position achieved by raising the head of the bed about 2 feet to provide better gas exchange in the lungs

systole—rhythmic contraction of the heart during which the blood is driven through the aorta and the pulmonary artery

ENHANCED OUTLINE

See text pages
_____

I. Congestive heart failure (CHF): circulatory congestion related to heart (pump) failure

A. Pathophysiology: frequently secondary to other health problems
1. Definitions
   a) Pump failure (heart failure): the inability of the heart to pump enough blood to meet the metabolic needs of the body
   b) Preload: the pressure of the blood that fills the ventricle during diastole
   c) Afterload: the resistance of the vessels into which the ventricle ejects blood during systole
   d) Stroke volume: the amount of blood ejected by the left ventricle on each contraction; depends on preload, ventricular contractility, and afterload
   e) Cardiac output: the amount of blood ejected by the heart each minute; depends on heart rate and stroke volume
   f) Cardiac reserve: the capacity of the heart to respond to an increased burden such as exercise, stress, or fever
   g) Ventricular dilation: increase in length of heart muscle (myocardial) fibers and enlargement of ventricle to increase cardiac output; increases oxygen demand of heart
   h) Ventricular hypertrophy: increased thickening of the ventricular wall to increase heart contractility; heart larger and heavier; heart works harder and requires more oxygen
2. Physiologic changes
   a) Changes in cardiac reserve: decreased, due to inability of heart to increase output in response to increased burden
   b) Cardiac compensation: In early chronic CHF, a decrease in cardiac reserve is offset by ventricular dilation, ventricular hypertrophy, and increased heart rate (tachycardia), which increase stroke volume.
   c) Tachycardia: Heart rate increases to increase cardiac output; with increasing heart rate, diastolic filling time decreases, eventually becoming counterproductive and leading to a decrease in cardiac output.

      d) Cardiac decompensation: Compensatory mechanisms fail to maintain adequate circulation, and symptoms of CHF become apparent with normal activity.
3. Left-sided heart failure: damage to left ventricle
      a) Sequence of events: Left ventricle hypertrophies and dilates; eventually, compensatory mechanisms fail; left ventricle is unable to eject full volume of blood; blood remains in dilated ventricle; left atrium dilates and hypertrophies; atrium fails to receive adequate blood from pulmonary veins, resulting in pulmonary congestion and pulmonary edema.
      b) Causes: congenital heart defects, hypertension, heart attack (myocardial infarction), both rheumatic fever and bacterial endocarditis affecting either the aortic valve or the mitral valve, and syphilis
4. Right-sided heart failure: due to increased pressure in pulmonary circulation system
      a) Sequence of events: Right ventricle tries to pump blood into congested lungs; pressure in lungs creates resistance to blood; blood backs up into venous circulation, causing congestion in gastrointestinal tract, liver, and kidney; peripheral edema develops.
      b) Causes: congenital heart defects and all causes of left-sided heart failure because it generally occurs after left-sided failure in response to increased pulmonary pressure
5. Mechanisms affecting fluid balance: fluid volume increases
      a) Stimulation of sympathetic nervous system: stroke volume increased; blood preferentially shunted to brain
      b) Renin-angiotensin-aldosterone system: decreased blood flow to kidneys results in renin production; produces angiotensin, which stimulates vasoconstriction (increases venous return to heart) and aldosterone production (increases sodium retention)
      c) Other hormones: Antidiuretic hormone (arginine vasopressin) increases water retention (increases preload).

B. Signs and symptoms
1. Changes in vital signs: increased pulse rate, increased respiration (tachypnea), increased blood pressure (hypertension)
2. Changes in fluid balance: fluid volume excess
      a) Pulmonary edema: left-sided heart failure; inhibited gas exchange in lungs; dry cough, wheezing, and moist rales; signs of overhydration
      b) Peripheral edema: right-sided failure; jugular vein distension, dependent pitting edema, rapid weight gain, enlarged liver, and fullness in abdomen
3. Changes in skin: bluish lips and nails (cyanosis) due to inadequate oxygen reaching tissues
4. Changes in laboratory results
      a) Serum sodium level normal or decreased due to dilution from retained water

      b) Serum potassium normal or decreased due to use of potassium-wasting diuretics and excess potassium loss with increased aldosterone

      c) Serum magnesium normal or decreased due to long-term use of potassium-wasting diuretics

      d) Serum chloride levels decreased when potassium-wasting diuretics are used for extended periods

      e) Metabolic acidosis due to decreased oxygen reaching cells and increased lactic acid

      f) Metabolic alkalosis due to long-term use of potassium-wasting diuretics

      g) Respiratory acidosis due to impaired gas exchange in lungs

C. Treatment and management: decrease workload of heart

  1. Diet: Restrict sodium intake, often in conjunction with bed rest; restrict water intake to prevent increase in edema.

  2. Diuretics: promote sodium and water excretion; decreases preload; may cause potassium imbalances

  3. Digitalization: achieving a serum level of digitalis (a cardiac glycoside) that has the appropriate physiologic effect (loading dose)

      a) Digitalis (e.g., digoxin, digitoxin, deslanoside) slows ventricular contractions and increases their strength.

      b) Digitalis toxicity is increased in the presence of certain electrolyte imbalances (see Nurse Alert, "Digitalis Toxicity").

  4. Venous vasodilators: nitroglycerine and isosorbide dinitrate reduce venous tone, causing venous pooling and decreased preload; used early in treatment to improve exercise tolerance and prolong life

  5. Other agents causing increased contractility: Norepinephrine, dopamine, and dobutamine all increase contractility but also increase arterial constriction (increased afterload); amrinone increases cardiac

---

! NURSE *ALERT* !

Digitalis Toxicity

Digitalis slows and strengthens the contractions of the heart. This potent drug is often given over protracted periods of time; cumulative effects may result in overdose because the difference between therapeutic and toxic levels is slight. The effect of digitalis is heightened by hypokalemia (most common), hypomagnesemia, hyponatremia, or hypercalcemia; toxicity may be precipitated by those electrolyte imbalances. The nurse must be alert for signs of digitalis toxicity (e.g., anorexia, nausea, vomiting, diarrhea, blurred vision, headache, confusion, depression, cardiac arrhythmias), especially when clients are being given potassium-wasting diuretics or IV calcium salts.

output—without tachycardia or arterial constriction—by altering calcium metabolism of heart cells.

D. Nursing process
   1. Nursing assessment: CHF often found in conjunction with other disease processes
     a) Assess baseline vital signs including heart sounds and lung sounds.
     b) Assess for signs of overhydration, which often indicate left-sided heart failure.
     c) Assess for signs of peripheral edema and abdominal fullness, which often indicate right-sided heart failure.
     d) Assess laboratory test values, especially serum potassium and sodium values.
   2. Nursing diagnoses
     a) Fluid volume excess related to failure to compensate for left-sided and/or right-sided heart failure
     b) Ineffective breathing patterns related to fluid in lungs secondary to cardiac decompensation
     c) Impaired tissue integrity secondary to edema in extremities
     d) Self-care deficit related to fatigue and breathlessness secondary to congestive heart failure
     e) Altered tissue perfusion related to cardiac insufficiency
     f) Activity intolerance related to cardiac insufficiency
   3. Nursing interventions
     a) Monitor for changes in vital signs and breathing patterns.
     b) Monitor response to diuretics by keeping very accurate fluid intake and output records.
     c) Check client in mornings for peripheral edema.
     d) Place client in Fowler's position to ease breathing.
     e) Educate client on food selection and seasoning for sodium-restricted diet.
     f) Educate client to eat high-potassium foods if potassium-wasting diuretics are prescribed.
     g) Provide skin care for areas where tissue integrity is impaired; encourage client to change position frequently.
     h) Assist client with self-care activities (bathing, feeding) as needed; educate family to help client with self-care.
     i) Monitor for signs of hypokalemia and/or digitalis toxicity.

II. Cardiopulmonary bypass during heart surgery

A. Fluid and electrolyte imbalances
   1. Massive expansion of the extracellular fluid (ECF) volume is needed to accommodate extracorporeal circulation.
     a) A weight gain of 5–15 lb is expected.
     b) ECF volume expansion can remain for up to 10 days postsurgery.
   2. Dilution-related deficits are common due to increased antidiuretic hormone production stimulated by cardiopulmonary bypass.

See text pages
_____

a) Hyponatremia
b) Hypokalemia: aggravated by urinary losses, especially if potassium-wasting diuretics have been used preoperatively
c) Hypomagnesemia: aggravated when chelating agents in banked blood bind magnesium

B. Management
   1. Use diuretics, as directed by physician, to reduce fluid volume.
   2. Replace electrolytes, as directed by physician.
   3. Before the operation, monitor for signs of digitalis toxicity the client who is taking digitalis.

See text pages
_____

III. Chronic obstructive pulmonary disease (COPD): disease associated with airway obstruction by narrowing of bronchioles

A. Pathophysiology: examples include emphysema, chronic bronchitis, bronchiectasis, and asthma; causes include alpha$_1$-antitrypsin deficiency (hereditary), chronic bacterial infection, air pollution, and inhaled chemical irritants; emphysema and chronic bronchitis most commonly related to tobacco smoking
   1. Morphologic changes: gas exchange reduced
      a) Thickening of bronchial walls: due to excess mucous secretion and submucosal edema; inhibits gas exchange
      b) Loss of elasticity of lung tissue: causes premature collapse of airways on expiration; dead air trapped
      c) Alveolar damage: distended alveoli, breakdown of alveolar septa; reduced gas exchange area; pulmonary hypertension
      d) Airway obstruction: edema, mucous plugs, narrowed bronchioles—especially during expiration
   2. Metabolic changes: Decreased oxygen reaches cells.
      a) Carbon dioxide retention: Respiratory acidosis results from poor gas exchange.
      b) Hypoxemia: Less oxygen diffuses into blood across alveolar capillary membrane due to thickening and reduced area.
      c) Increase in red blood cells: an attempt to compensate for hypoxemia
      d) Pulmonary hypertension: due to destruction of pulmonary capillary bed; leads to right-sided heart failure
      e) Alpha$_1$-antitrypsin deficiency: genetic defect resulting in destruction of lung tissue and emphysema

B. Signs and symptoms
   1. Changes in vital signs: increased blood pressure and pulse rate; labored respirations with prolonged expiration
   2. Other pulmonary changes: cough that produces mucus; shortness of breath with exertion (early) or without significant exertion (late)

3. Other changes: barrel-shaped chest, cyanosis, clubbing of nails, chronic fatigue
4. Changes in arterial blood gases
   a) pH <7.35
   b) $PaCO_2$ >45 mm Hg
   c) HCO_3 >26 mEq/L
   d) PaO_2 <80 mm Hg (normal 80–110 mm Hg)
   e) BE >+2 (when respiratory acidosis exists with metabolic compensation)
5. Changes in other laboratory values
   a) Increased hemoglobin and hematocrit
   b) Low to normal serum potassium
   c) Normal to slightly increased serum sodium

C. Treatment and management
1. Low-flow oxygen: 1–2 liters per minute with nasal cannula or 24%–28% with Venturi mask; too much oxygen depresses respiratory drive
2. Hydration: increasing fluid intake to 3–4 liters/day helps liquefy secretions in lungs; contraindicated if client has CHF
3. Bronchodilators: isoproterenol (Isuprel), metaproterenol sulfate (Alupent), terbutaline sulfate (Brethine), aminophylline, and theophylline products; all dilate bronchioles, promote expectoration of mucus, and improve ventilation; administered through nebulizers, IV, or orally
4. Antibiotics: IV or orally for respiratory infection
5. Chest physiotherapy: chest clapping (loosens mucus), positioning for postural drainage (uses gravity to help drain diseased areas of lungs), diaphragmatic breathing (improves alveolar ventilation), and pursed-lip breathing (prevents airway collapse)
6. Exercise: walking and using stationary bicycle; improves respiratory status and general health
7. Relaxation techniques: help prevent panic due to dyspnea

D. Nursing process
1. Nursing assessment
   a) Obtain client history of respiratory-related problems.
   b) Assess vital signs and lung sounds.
   c) Assess arterial blood gas readings.
2. Nursing diagnoses
   a) Impaired gas exchange related to alveolar damage and narrowed bronchioles
   b) Ineffective airway clearance related to mucous secretions and narrowed bronchioles
   c) Activity intolerance related to breathlessness and fatigue
   d) Anxiety related to breathlessness
   e) Altered tissue perfusion related to hypoxemia secondary to chronic obstructive pulmonary disease
   f) Impaired physical mobility related to breathlessness
3. Nursing interventions
   a) Monitor vital signs, lung sounds, arterial blood gases, and fluid status.
   b) Assist with administration of oxygen and bronchodilators.

I. Congestive heart failure (CHF)	II. Cardiopulmonary bypass during heart surgery	III. Chronic obstructive pulmonary disease (COPD)

c) Perform chest clapping while client is in appropriate postural drainage position.
d) Instruct client in breathing exercises and bronchodilator use.
e) Explain relaxation techniques.
f) Educate and support family members in assisting client with chest physiotherapy.

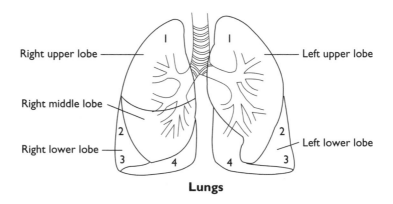

Right upper lobe — Left upper lobe
Right middle lobe —
Right lower lobe — Left lower lobe

Lungs

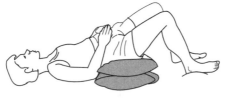

1. Upper lobes, anterior

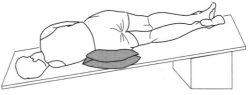

3. Lower lobes, lateral

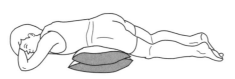

2. Lower lobes, superior

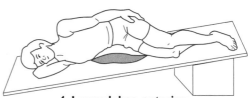

4. Lower lobes, anterior

Figure 9–1
Positioning for Postural Drainage

1. A 68-year-old client is at risk for left ventricular failure due to prolonged high blood pressure. The nurse should monitor the client for:
   a. Pitting pedal edema.
   b. Loss of appetite.
   c. Chronic nonproductive cough.
   d. Excessive urine output.

2. An 87-year-old client has chronic congestive heart failure. To assess for exacerbation of the congestive heart failure, the nurse should assess the client for:
   a. Nocturia.
   b. Slow venous return after elevation of hands.
   c. Narrowed pulse pressure.
   d. Bradycardia.

3. Which of the following nursing diagnoses is most appropriate for the client with congestive heart failure?
   a. Fluid volume deficit related to deficient ADH production
   b. Activity intolerance related to fatigue and dyspnea
   c. Risk for injury related to low blood pressure
   d. Diarrhea related to third spacing of fluid in intestines

4. A 75-year-old client is admitted with acute pulmonary edema. In which position should the nurse place the client?
   a. Left lateral Sims
   b. Supine with legs elevated
   c. Trendelenburg
   d. High Fowler's

5. A client is admitted in acute congestive heart failure. Digoxin is ordered. Which of the following outcomes indicates that digoxin is having a therapeutic effect?
   a. Increased jugular venous pressure
   b. Increased heart rate
   c. Increased urine output
   d. Increased respiratory rate

6. A client is admitted to the cardiac care unit after receiving cardiopulmonary resuscitation during a cardiac arrest. The client's serum potassium on admission is 5.8 mEq/L. Which of the following changes in the client's electrocardiogram (ECG) is the nurse most likely to find?
   a. Depressed S-T segment
   b. Flattened T wave
   c. Appearance of U waves
   d. Absence of P waves

7. A client required cardiopulmonary bypass during cardiac surgery. During the immediate postoperative period, the nurse should expect to find:
   a. Loss of 5–10 lb.
   b. Low serum sodium.
   c. Elevated serum potassium.
   d. Poor skin turgor.

8. A 60-year-old client has emphysema, which is being treated with bronchodilators and steroids. Which of the following lab test results should the nurse expect for this client?
   a. Low serum bicarbonate
   b. High hemoglobin
   c. Low serum sodium
   d. High serum potassium

9. A 50-year-old client is chronically short of breath due to chronic obstructive pulmonary disease (COPD). Which of the following symptoms is the nurse most likely to observe in this client?
   a. Warm, flushed skin
   b. Numbness of fingers and toes
   c. Dull headache
   d. Blurred vision

10. A 67-year-old client has severe COPD. Which of the following nursing diagnoses is most likely to be appropriate for this client?

a. High risk for fluid volume excess, peripheral edema, related to right ventricular failure

b. Alteration in acid-base balance, respiratory alkalosis, related to rapid respiratory rate

c. Risk for injury related to bone demineralization due to hypocalcemia

d. Alteration in urinary elimination, polyuria, related to a steroid-induced increase in sodium excretion

11. A 55-year-old client who has COPD experiences carbon dioxide (CO_2) retention. To promote deep breathing and mobilize secretions, the physician prescribes a daily walk. The nurse should advise the client to plan to walk:

a. Immediately before going to bed.
b. Late in the afternoon.
c. Immediately after lunch.
d. Before breakfast.

12. A client who has chronic emphysema is dyspneic and cyanotic. To improve the client's breathing pattern, the nurse should:

a. Limit the client's fluid intake to 1500 ml/day.
b. Administer oxygen (O_2) via a nonrebreathing mask.
c. Place the client in semi-Fowler's position.
d. Teach the client pursed-lip breathing.

ANSWERS

1. **Correct answer is c.** Left ventricular failure increases the pressure in pulmonary vessels, causing pulmonary edema, which stimulates a hacking nonproductive cough.

a. Pedal edema develops when the right ventricle fails. It would not be an early sign of left ventricular failure.
b. Engorgement of gastrointestinal (GI) vessels and liver enlargement, which occur in right ventricular failure, cause anorexia.
d. Urine output is reduced in both left and right ventricular failure and is due to

reduced renal perfusion when cardiac output decreases.

2. **Correct answer is a.** Nocturia is associated with worsening of congestive heart failure, because cardiac output improves with rest and recumbent position. As cardiac output improves, renal vasoconstriction decreases—improving glomerular filtration—so urine output increases.

b and c. Slowed venous return and narrowed pulse pressure are signs of hypovolemia. Hypervolemia occurs with congestive heart failure and is due to elevated aldosterone levels and reduced renal perfusion.
d. Congestive heart failure produces tachycardia as the heart attempts to compensate for decreased cardiac output by increasing the heart rate.

3. **Correct answer is b.** Fatigue occurs due to tissue hypoxia when cardiac output is reduced. Pulmonary edema causes dyspnea with exertion.

a. Fluid volume excess is more likely. Elevated renin levels in congestive heart failure increase production of aldosterone, resulting in retention of sodium and fluid.
c. High blood pressure due to hypervolemia is more likely.
d. Congestive heart failure does not cause third spacing of fluid in the intestines. Constipation is more likely and would be due to shifting of circulation away from the GI tract to maintain the blood supply to the heart and brain.

4. **Correct answer is d.** Gravity keeps fluid at the base of the lungs, permitting effective gas exchange in the upper portions of the lung. High Fowler's position also reduces venous return, thereby lowering cardiac preload, which is therapeutic in congestive heart failure.

a, b, and c. All of these positions increase venous return, which raises cardiac preload. They also permit fluid to spread throughout the lungs, impairing gas exchange.

5. **Correct answer is c.** Fluid retention is a compensatory mechanism triggered by low cardiac output. As cardiac output improves due to improved contractility in response to digoxin, diuresis occurs.

a. In congestive heart failure, jugular venous pressure is elevated due to hypervolemia. Reduced jugular venous pressure would be a therapeutic effect of digoxin.
b. Digoxin slows the heart rate. Bradycardia is a common side effect.
d. Dyspnea produces rapid, shallow respirations. A reduced respiratory rate would reflect therapeutic effects of digoxin.

6. **Correct answer is d.** Hyperkalemia produces prolonged P-R intervals, tall peaked T waves, widened QRS complexes, and absence of P waves.

a, b, and **c.** All are changes associated with hypokalemia.

7. **Correct answer is b.** Dilutional hyponatremia often occurs because cardiopulmonary bypass raises ADH levels more than does surgery alone, so more water than sodium is retained.

a. A weight gain of 5–15 lb is expected due to the massive extracellular volume expansion required for cardiopulmonary bypass.
c. Hypokalemia occurs due to hemodilution and shifting of potassium into cells.
d. Poor skin turgor is associated with fluid volume deficit. After cardiopulmonary bypass, fluid volume excess occurs.

8. **Correct answer is b.** Hemoglobin increases in response to chronic hypoxemia. More hemoglobin can carry more oxygen.

a. Carbon dioxide (CO_2) retention in emphysema produces acidosis. Bicarbonate (HCO_3) is retained to compensate, so HCO_3 levels are likely to be elevated.
c. Usually, sodium level remains normal with emphysema, but it may be slightly elevated. Hyponatremia is unlikely.

d. Hypokalemia is likely. Steroids promote potassium loss. Dietary intake may be reduced due to breathlessness.

9. **Correct answer is c.** Dull headache is a common symptom of chronic respiratory acidosis.

a. Warm, flushed skin occurs in acute respiratory acidosis, because the body has no time to compensate for the elevated CO_2 levels.
b and **d.** These are symptoms of alkalosis.

10. **Correct answer is a.** Right ventricular failure is a common complication of severe COPD. Increased venous hydrostatic pressure due to right ventricular failure produces peripheral edema.

b. Collapse of bronchiolar lumina on expiration and the retention of respiratory secretions reduce CO_2 excretion, leading to respiratory acidosis.
c. Hypocalcemia can cause bone demineralization, thereby increasing the risk for injury. However, calcium balance is not usually altered by COPD.
d. Steroids increase potassium excretion and produce sodium and fluid retention. The resultant decrease in renal fluid excretion produces oliguria.

11. **Correct answer is b.** Lungs are best able to expand when the stomach is empty. Once the client has been awake and sitting up, retention of secretions is reduced and gas exchange will be better. This reduces the fatigue that occurs with hypoxia.

a. Exercise before bed stimulates the sympathetic nervous system, promoting wakefulness. Because insomnia is a side effect of bronchodilators used to treat COPD, any action that promotes wakefulness at night should be avoided.
c. After meals, energy is needed for digestion. Activity intolerance worsens if exercise is attempted at that time.
d. Secretions are retained during sleep. Until they are mobilized, gas exchange is impaired and activity intolerance is worse.

12. **Correct answer is d.** Pursed-lip breathing increases airway pressure during expiration, allowing trapped air to be expelled and leaving more space for inspired air, which provides more oxygen.

a. Fluids should be forced to liquefy secretions so that secretions can be more easily expectorated. This relieves airway obstruction, thereby reducing air trapping.

b. Nonrebreathing masks are contraindicated, because they deliver high oxygen concentrations. The client's chronic high CO_2 level eliminates the brain's normal stimulus to breathe (rising CO_2 level). The client depends on hypoxia to stimulate respirations. Raising the PaO_2 (partial pressure of oxygen in arterial blood) level too high would eliminate the drive to breathe.

c. The client needs to be in orthopneic position (sitting, and leaning slightly forward) to relieve dyspnea and promote lung expansion.

10

Renal Failure

NURSING HIGHLIGHTS

1. Acute renal failure is usually reversible if treated in time; chronic renal failure is irreversible.
2. Signs and symptoms appear almost immediately in acute renal failure; chronic renal failure is insidious, with symptoms appearing only after renal failure is entrenched.
3. Compensation occurs with chronic renal failure, thereby delaying signs, symptoms, and laboratory indications of the condition.

GLOSSARY

azotemia—buildup of nitrogenous waste products such as urea in the blood as indicated by elevated blood urea nitrogen (BUN) and serum creatinine

dialysate—iso-osmolar solution used in dialysis that contains calcium chloride, magnesium chloride, potassium chloride, sodium chloride, and either sodium acetate or bicarbonate; glucose may be added to make the dialysate hyperosmolar in peritoneal dialysis

dialysis—process of filtering nitrogenous wastes and excess fluids through a semipermeable membrane

ultrafiltration—enhancement of the movement of fluids across a semipermeable membrane by means of an induced pressure gradient

uremic syndrome—toxic condition affecting all organ systems and caused by failure of the kidneys to excrete nitrogenous waste products

ENHANCED OUTLINE

See text pages

I. Pathophysiology and etiology: failure to regulate blood pressure, detoxify and eliminate waste products, regulate erythropoiesis (red blood cell formation), synthesize prostaglandin, metabolize vitamin D, and regulate volume, concentration, and pH of blood; results in metabolic, biochemical, fluid, electrolyte, and acid-base abnormalities

A. Acute renal failure (ARF): abrupt, reversible cessation of renal function, resulting in azotemia and uremic syndrome

    1. Types of ARF

        a) Prerenal: decreased perfusion; hypovolemia, cardiac failure, and vascular embolism; potentially reversible

        b) Postrenal: obstruction; ureteral fibrosis, calculi (stones), clots, and neoplasms; potentially reversible

        c) Parenchymal: tissue damage; glomerulonephritis, renal vascular disease, acute tubular necrosis, and toxic hemolysis; may not be reversible

    2. Phases of ARF

        a) Initial phase (onset)

            (1) Phase begins with precipitating tissue insult (e.g., hemorrhage, ureteral blockage, acute disease).

            (2) Phase ends when signs of azotemia and oliguria appear.

            (3) Initial phase normally lasts 0–2 days.

            (4) During the period, renal blood flow diminishes to 25% of normal, filtration clearance diminishes to 10% of normal, and urine output diminishes to 20% of normal.

        b) Oliguric/anuric phase (anuria rarely occurs)

            (1) Urine output decreases further to less than 400 ml/day (5% of normal).

(2) BUN and serum creatinine are substantially elevated.

(3) Renal blood flow remains at 25% of normal; filtration clearance remains at 10% of normal.

(4) Phase lasts 8–14 days; the longer this phase lasts, the greater the probability of serious fluid, electrolyte, and metabolic complications.

(5) Dialysis is begun in this stage.

   c) Diuretic phase

(1) Phase is initiated by sudden increase in urine output (at least 1500 ml/day).

(2) Serum laboratory values stop rising and then later fall.

(3) Kidney is unable to concentrate urine; fluid and electrolytes are lost; client has high risk of dehydration.

(4) Phase lasts 10 or more days.

   d) Recovery phase (convalescence)

(1) Serum laboratory values stabilize.

(2) Normal or optimal kidney function is restored.

(3) Phase can last months.

B. Chronic renal failure (CRF): progressive, insidious, irreversible renal damage that results in metabolic, fluid, electrolyte, and acid-base imbalances

  1. Causes of CRF

   a) Congenital disorders: fused kidney, displaced kidney, hypoplastic kidney, hereditary nephritis, polycystic kidney disease, and medullary cystic kidney disease

   b) Systemic diseases: diabetes mellitus (common), diabetes insipidus, systemic lupus erythematosus, scleroderma, amyloidosis, primary hyperparathyroidism, and hypertension

   c) Tubular disorders: renal tubular acidosis and chronic electrolyte imbalances (e.g., hypercalcemic nephropathy, hypokalemic nephropathy)

   d) Glomerular disorders: glomerulonephritis and nephrotic syndrome

   e) Obstructive disorders: nephrolithiasis and retroperitoneal fibrosis

   f) Infectious diseases: tuberculosis and pyelonephritis

   g) Neoplastic diseases: lymphoma and multiple myeloma

  2. Stages of CRF

   a) Stage I: diminished renal reserve

(1) Mild reduction in renal function; 40%–70% of normal

(2) No obvious symptoms; client usually unaware of condition

   b) Stage II: renal insufficiency

(1) Kidney function is further reduced to 20%–40% of normal.

(2) Glomerular filtration rate, ability to concentrate urine, and hormone production are diminished.

(3) BUN and serum creatinine values increase.

(4) Signs and symptoms such as polyuria, anemia, and azotemia become noticeable, especially if other kidney stressors (e.g., dehydration) are present.

    c) Stage III: end-stage renal disease (ESRD)
      (1) Renal function is less than 15% of normal.
      (2) Kidney is unable to maintain excretory, regulatory, or hormonal functions.
      (3) BUN and serum creatinine are dramatically elevated and continue to rise.
      (4) Anemia, azotemia, and hyperuricemia are present.
      (5) Oliguria develops with high urine osmolality and fluid volume excess.
      (6) Electrolyte imbalances include hyperphosphatemia, hypocalcemia, metabolic acidosis, and hyperkalemia.
      (7) Uremic syndrome develops: Functional deterioration of renal system approaches completion; every organ system is affected.
      (8) 100% mortality occurs unless dialysis begins.

II. Fluid and electrolyte imbalances

See text pages

A. Fluid volume imbalances
    1. Fluid volume excess: appears in oliguric stage of ARF and end-stage CRF; urine output falls; kidney fails to dilute and excrete urine
    2. Fluid volume deficit: appears in diuretic stage of ARF; often accompanied by electrolyte imbalances

B. Electrolyte imbalances
    1. Sodium imbalances
      a) Hypernatremia: decreased intravascular volume, increased sodium reabsorption due to increased aldosterone secretion
      b) Hyponatremia: excessive loss of electrolytes in diuretic phase of ARF; metabolic acidosis also shifts sodium into cells
    2. Potassium imbalances
      a) Hyperkalemia: significant in both ARF and CRF, but more dangerous in ARF; decreased glomerular filtration rate and excretion; cellular injury releases potassium; metabolic acidosis shifts potassium out of cells
      b) Hypokalemia: excessive potassium loss during diuretic phase of ARF; excessive loss of gastric secretions; excessive dialysis; renal tubular acidosis, resulting in potassium excretion
    3. Hypocalcemia: occurs in both ARF and CRF
      a) Accompanies phosphate retention; inverse relationship between phosphate and calcium
      b) Decreased calcium absorbed from intestine because vitamin D activity impaired

      c) Results in deposition of calcium phosphate in soft tissues

    4. Hyperphosphatemia: occurs in both ARF and CRF

      a) Decreased glomerular filtration rate and renal tubule function result in impaired excretion.

      b) Phosphate shifts from cells to extracellular fluid due to cell lysis.

      c) Metabolic acidosis inhibits formation of phosphate salts for excretion.

    5. Chloride and magnesium: imbalances normally clinically insignificant

C. Acid-base imbalances: metabolic acidosis

    1. Condition occurs in both ARF and CRF, but more compensation occurs in CRF.

    2. Hydrogen ions and metabolic acids are not excreted.

    3. Less bicarbonate is resorbed by damaged nephrons.

    4. Lactic acid forms due to tissue hypoxia.

    5. Fat breaks down, forming ketone acids.

III. Signs and symptoms: unless noted, related to uremic toxins (see chapters 2, 3, and 4 for signs and symptoms of specific fluid, electrolyte, and acid-base imbalances)

See text pages
_____

A. Neurologic: slow neural conduction, changes in thought process and level of consciousness, and seizures

B. Cardiovascular: pericarditis, hypertension and congestive heart failure (fluid volume excess), and arrhythmias (electrolyte imbalances)

C. Respiratory: pulmonary edema (fluid volume excess) and pneumonia (excessive bronchial secretions, reduced immune response)

D. Gastrointestinal: ulcers, indigestion, and uremic halitosis

E. Hematologic: reduced immune response, impaired coagulation of blood due to decreased platelet survival, and anemia (erythropoietin production interrupted, decreased red blood cell count)

F. Musculoskeletal (CRF): calcification of soft tissue and brittle bones (calcium and phosphorus imbalance)

G. Endocrine: secondary hyperparathyroidism (calcium and phosphorus imbalance)

H. Integumentary: dry, bronzed skin

IV. Treatment and management: dialysis

See text pages
_____

A. Continuous renal replacement therapy (CRRT): most effective for ARF; conducted only in intensive care unit (ICU)

    1. Filtration process: continuous

      a) Hemofilter (porous blood filter with semipermeable membrane) is positioned in circulatory loop created outside the body; this requires vein and artery cannulization.

       b) Client's mean arterial pressure (MAP) drives filtration process.

       c) Three types of filtration exist—slow continuous ultrafiltration (SCUF), continuous arteriovenous hemofiltration (CAVH), and continuous arteriovenous hemodialysis (CAVHD).

2. Indications for CRRT

       a) CRF, with client unable to tolerate other dialysis due to pulmonary edema, congestive heart failure, gastrointestinal bleeding, or cardiogenic shock

       b) ARF, with client hemodynamically unstable and unable to tolerate either hemodialysis or peritoneal dialysis (e.g., cardiac bypass surgery, myocardial infarction, sepsis)

       c) ARF, with client who requires daily removal of uremic toxins and fluid and electrolyte adjustments because of high catabolic rate

       d) Oliguria, with client who needs large volume of IV fluids or total parenteral nutrition

3. Advantages of CRRT: rapid fluid removal, electrolytes easily adjusted, does not require stable cardiovascular or hemodynamic status, cost-effective

4. Disadvantages of CRRT: must be done in ICU setting, requires vascular access, risk of blood clotting, risk of dehydration

B. Hemodialysis

1. Filtration process: takes 3–4 hours

       a) Heated iso-osmolar dialysate solution is delivered to artificial kidney.

       b) Artificial kidney is essentially a semipermeable membrane; designs include flat plate and hollow fiber.

       c) Large vein is catheterized, and client's blood is pumped through artificial kidney.

       d) Uremic waste and excess water move from blood across semipermeable membrane and into dialysate; ultrafiltration occurs.

2. Advantages of hemodialysis: fluid, uremic wastes, and toxic drugs removed rapidly; electrolyte imbalances corrected quickly; can be used when abdominal trauma exists; used for ARF or CRF

3. Disadvantages of hemodialysis: high cost, requires large doses of heparin—high risk of clotting, requires complex equipment, risk of overly rapid fluid and electrolyte shifts (see Nurse Alert, "Disequilibrium Syndrome"), poorly tolerated by clients with cardiovascular disease

C. Peritoneal dialysis

1. Filtration process: Time varies for acute and chronic conditions.

       a) Sterile hyperosmolar dialysate/glucose solution is infused into peritoneal cavity by gravity flow (glucose used to make solution hyperosmolar).

       b) Peritoneum acts as semipermeable membrane.

Disequilibrium Syndrome

Disequilibrium syndrome consists of a group of signs and symptoms thought to be caused by cerebral edema and/or increased pressure from cerebrospinal fluid related to rapid changes in serum osmolality. The nurse should monitor clients undergoing hemodialysis, especially the first few times, for the following:

- Restlessness
- Nausea
- Hypertension
- Confusion
- Muscle twitching
- Coma

- Headache
- Vomiting
- Increased intracranial pressure
- Psychiatric problems
- Convulsions

    c) Ultrafiltration occurs because of osmotic pressure gradient between blood and hyperosmolar dialysate; waste moves across peritoneum and into dialysate.

    d) Gravity flow is used to remove dialysate from peritoneal cavity.

2. Advantages of peritoneal dialysis: requires no direct access to vascular system, requires little heparin—low risk of clotting, minimal

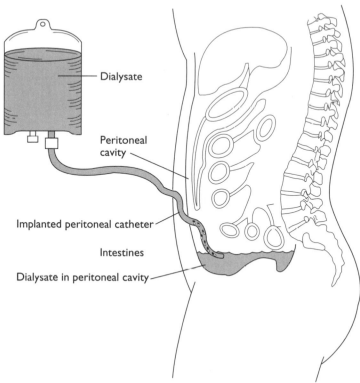

Figure 10–1
Peritoneal Dialysis

stress for clients with cardiovascular disease, cost-effective, used for ARF or CRF
   3. Disadvantages of peritoneal dialysis: fluids, electrolytes, and wastes removed slowly; toxic drugs not removed efficiently; frequent treatments (3 or 4 times daily); high risk of peritonitis; not used for clients with abdominal trauma or surgery

V. Nursing process

A. Nursing assessment
   1. Assess client's history relative to previous renal-related problems, systemic diseases, familial predisposition to renal problems, and drug history.
   2. Assess baseline vital signs and laboratory test values.
   3. Assess fluid intake and output; assess for signs of fluid volume imbalances.
   4. Assess for signs of specific electrolyte imbalances.

B. Nursing diagnoses: many collaborative diagnoses with physician
   1. Fluid volume excess related to fluid retention secondary to renal failure
   2. Fluid volume deficit related to inappropriate dialysis
   3. Altered urinary output related to kidney impairment
   4. High risk for infection related to cannulization for hemodialysis or to insertion of catheter for peritoneal dialysis

C. Nursing interventions
   1. Monitor fluid intake and output along with daily weight and girth changes.
   2. Monitor vital signs and laboratory test values; note electrolyte imbalances.
   3. Assist as needed with dialysis procedures.
   4. Use aseptic techniques to care for cannulas and catheters.

1. A client who is receiving tobramycin (Nebcin) needs to be observed for acute renal failure (ARF). To promptly detect the onset of ARF, the nurse should monitor the client for:

   a. Elevated BUN and creatinine.
   b. Decreased urine osmolality.
   c. Proteinuria.
   d. Elevated serum potassium.

2. A 50-year-old client has end-stage renal disease (ESRD). Lab results include: serum potassium = 6.5 mEq/L, serum calcium = 8.3 mg/dl, arterial pH = 7.31, and serum creatinine = 8.5 mg/dl. It is most important for the nurse to carefully monitor this client for:

   a. Kussmaul breathing.
   b. Tetany.
   c. Cardiac arrhythmias.
   d. Paralytic ileus.

3. A client with ESRD is having peritoneal dialysis with an infusion of 2000 ml of dialysate. After a 4-hour dwell time, 1600 ml of solution returns. The nurse should assess the client for:

   a. Seizures.
   b. Crackles in the lung bases.
   c. Flaccid paralysis of the legs.
   d. Loss of deep-tendon reflexes.

4. A client is in the oliguric phase of ARF. Which nursing diagnosis is most likely to be appropriate for this client?

   a. Constipation related to slow peristalsis secondary to hypokalemia
   b. Impaired physical mobility related to muscle weakness secondary to hypercalcemia
   c. Risk for injury related to light-headedness secondary to alkalosis
   d. Impaired gas exchange related to pulmonary edema secondary to hypervolemia

5. A client with chronic renal failure (CRF) has a serum phosphorus of 9.5 mg/dl and a serum calcium of 8.2 mg/dl. Which of the following nursing diagnoses describes the complication for which this client is at greatest risk based on those electrolyte levels?

   a. Risk for impaired skin integrity related to pruritis
   b. Risk for infection related to immune system suppression
   c. Diarrhea related to gastrointestinal tract hypermotility
   d. Fatigue related to decreased production of red blood cells

6. A 25-year-old client is in the diuretic phase of ARF. The client's urine output is 2500 ml/day. The nursing care plan should include:

   a. Providing high-protein snacks.
   b. Elevating the head of the bed.
   c. Giving mouth care frequently.
   d. Limiting intake of fruit juices.

7. A client has CRF. Creatinine clearance is 10 mg/minute, and serum creatinine is 3.5 mg/dl. The client's nursing care plan should include:

   a. Encouraging the client to drink 2–3 liters of fluid daily.
   b. Teaching the client to increase intake of milk and cheeses.
   c. Advising the client to drink more citrus juices.
   d. Suggesting that the client eat high-protein snacks.

8. A client with ARF is started on hemodialysis. The nurse must observe this client for:

   a. Dyspnea and coughing.
   b. Agitation and muscle twitching.
   c. Weakness and lethargy.
   d. Slow, shallow breathing.

9. A client develops ARF after cardiac surgery. Continuous renal replacement therapy (CRRT) is initiated. The nurse should carefully monitor the client for:

   a. Hyperkalemia.
   b. Dilutional hyponatremia.
   c. Fluid volume deficit.
   d. Respiratory alkalosis.

10. A client is in the oliguric stage of ARF. Serum potassium is 6.2 mEq/L. IV D_5W with insulin is ordered. The nurse can explain to the client that this therapy will:

    a. Increase excretion of potassium in urine due to osmotic diuresis.
    b. Shift potassium into cells, which lowers serum levels.
    c. Produce osmotic diarrhea with potassium loss in stools.
    d. Increase utilization of potassium by speeding up cellular metabolism.

11. A client has CRF. Aluminum hydroxide (Amphojel) 30 ml PO QID is ordered. The nurse recognizes that this therapy is effective if the client has which of the following outcomes?

    a. Urine output = 1800 ml/day
    b. Serum potassium = 4.5 mEq/L
    c. Blood pH = 7.35
    d. Serum phosphorus = 4.0 mg/dl

12. A client with ESRD is short of breath and has distended neck veins. Peritoneal dialysis is initiated with 4.25% dextrose dialysate for the first exchange. The intended outcome of using such a dialysate solution is:

    a. Correction of hypoglycemia.
    b. Normalization of serum sodium.
    c. Prevention of cardiac arrhythmias.
    d. Rapid removal of excess fluid.

ANSWERS

1. **Correct answer is a.** Elevated BUN (blood urea nitrogen) and creatinine are early signs of ARF.

   b. Urine osmolality decreases in the diuretic phase of ARF.
   c. Proteinuria and hematuria are early signs of CRF. In ARF, BUN and creatinine would rise first.
   d. Serum potassium rises during the oliguric phase, but BUN and creatinine rise first.

2. **Correct answer is c.** Hypocalcemia potentiates the adverse effects of hyperkalemia on the heart, including arrhythmias. Metabolic acidosis—common with ESRD—further increases the risk.

   a. Rapid, deep respirations (Kussmaul breathing) are a compensatory mechanism, enabling the client to reduce blood acidity via excretion of carbon dioxide.
   b. Tetany may occur with hypocalcemia. It is not life threatening; cardiac arrhythmias are.
   d. Paralytic ileus occurs with hypokalemia. This client is hyperkalemic.

3. **Correct answer is b.** Retained dialysate can be absorbed, producing hypervolemia. Symptoms of pulmonary edema, including crackles at the lung bases, result.

   a. Seizures occur with intracellular fluid volume excess. The client with ESRD retains large amounts of electrolytes, which would prevent fluid from shifting to the intracellular space.
   c. This is a sign of hyperkalemia. Retained dialysate would reduce serum potassium, so new signs of hyperkalemia would not be expected to appear.
   d. This is a sign of hypermagnesemia. Retained dialysate would reduce serum magnesium, so new signs of hypermagnesemia would not be expected.

4. **Correct answer is d.** In the oliguric phase, fluid is retained because the kidneys cannot dilute urine. Pulmonary edema due to hypervolemia may develop.

   a. During the oliguric phase, potassium is retained. This nursing diagnosis is appropriate for the diuretic phase.

b. In ARF, phosphate is retained. Calcium levels decrease as phosphate levels rise.

c. In ARF, acidosis is most common. The kidneys cannot resorb bicarbonate, and therefore the acid by-products of metabolism are not excreted.

5. **Correct answer is a.** High phosphorus and low calcium in combination promote deposition of calcium phosphate crystals in the skin, thereby producing intense itching.

   b. Uremic toxins decrease neutrophil activity and increase infection risk. This is not a result of calcium or phosphorus imbalance.
   c. This nursing diagnosis is related to hyperkalemia. Neither increased phosphorus nor decreased calcium causes diarrhea.
   d. This nursing diagnosis is related to decreased erythropoietin production and uremic toxins, which reduce red blood cell survival time. It is not related to calcium or phosphorus balance.

6. **Correct answer is c.** During the diuretic phase, fluid volume deficit often develops and mucous membranes become dry and sticky. Frequent mouth care prevents damage to the mucous membranes and increases comfort.

   a. Acid by-products from protein contribute to metabolic acidosis. Protein is usually restricted in ARF.
   b. This would be appropriate to reduce dyspnea due to pulmonary edema that might develop in the oliguric phase. In the diuretic phase, hypovolemia occurs. Keeping the head low helps maintain cerebral perfusion.
   d. During the diuretic phase, potassium is lost and hypokalemia may develop. Fruit juices tend to be high in potassium and would be restricted in the oliguric phase. They would be permitted in the diuretic phase.

7. **Correct answer is a.** In the renal insufficiency stage, fluids are encouraged to help

excrete wastes, because the kidneys do not function efficiently.

   b. Increased calcium intake would be appropriate. However, cheeses are high in sodium and milk is high in phosphorus. These electrolytes need to be limited.
   c. Citrus juices are high in potassium. Because hyperkalemia is a risk, the client should not increase intake of potassium.
   d. Protein metabolism produces acid waste products, thereby increasing the risk for metabolic acidosis. Dietary protein may be restricted in CRF.

8. **Correct answer is b.** Agitation and muscle twitching are signs of disequilibrium syndrome, which occurs due to the rapid shifting of fluids and electrolytes during hemodialysis.

   a. Dyspnea and coughing are signs of pulmonary edema related to hypervolemia. Hemodialysis is more likely to cause hypovolemia.
   c. Weakness and lethargy are signs of hypercalcemia. Hemodialysis would not raise serum calcium levels above normal unless calcium were added to the dialysate.
   d. Slow, shallow breathing would reflect hypochloremia. The chloride level in dialysate resembles that in plasma, so hypochloremia is unlikely.

9. **Correct answer is c.** The risk for dehydration and hypovolemia is increased with CRRT because fluid is rapidly removed.

   a. CRRT helps to reduce serum potassium, which is usually elevated during the oliguric phase of ARF.
   b. Fluid is removed, not added, by CRRT. Serum sodium is more likely to rise than to fall.
   d. Respiratory alkalosis occurs with hyperventilation. CRRT does not affect respiratory function the way peritoneal dialysis would.

10. **Correct answer is b.** Potassium is shifted into cells with glucose. Insulin increases glucose transport into cells, thus enhancing potassium movement into cells and reducing serum potassium.

    a. Osmotic diuresis occurs when blood glucose is elevated. Insulin reduces blood glucose, so osmotic diuresis is unlikely.
    c. This describes the effect of cation exchange resins, such as sodium polystyrene sulfonate (Kayexalate).
    d. Potassium is not utilized in cellular metabolism. Insulin and glucose do not speed cellular metabolism.

11. **Correct answer is d.** The aluminum in Amphojel binds phosphates in the intestines so they are excreted in the stool.

    a, b, and **c.** Amphojel has no therapeutic effect on urine output, potassium levels, or acid-base balance. It is used as a phosphate binder in renal disease.

12. **Correct answer is d.** A 4.5% dialysate solution has a high osmolality, which produces ultrafiltration, thereby shifting fluid rapidly into the abdomen, to be removed when the dialysate is drained.

    a. Dextrose from the dialysate does not cross the peritoneal membrane to enter circulation rapidly enough to affect blood glucose. IV glucose would be used to correct hypoglycemia.
    b and **c.** An advantage of peritoneal dialysis is that electrolyte levels are altered slowly. Cardiac arrhythmias occur with hyperkalemia, so answer *c* would reflect reduction of potassium.

11

Clinical Oncology

NURSING HIGHLIGHTS

1. Fluid and electrolyte imbalances may be the first clinical symptoms of undiagnosed cancer.
2. General deterioration involving many organ systems is common in clients with advanced cancer and must be considered in any attempt to improve fluid and electrolyte imbalances.

GLOSSARY

cancer—a group of diseases characterized by abnormal and uncontrolled cell growth, in which malignant cells invade normal tissues and spread to distant locations in the body

ENHANCED OUTLINE

See text pages

I. Pathophysiology

A. Characteristics of cancer cells: uncontrolled and abnormal growth; able to invade and reorganize normal tissue; more primitive (anaplastic) than normal cells; tend to produce inappropriate proteins, enzymes, or hormones; unresponsive to normal regulatory mechanisms

B. Types of cancer cells: individual solid tumors (e.g., carcinoma, sarcoma); abnormal cells in lymph nodes (lymphoma) or bone marrow (leukemia) that are carried throughout the body

See text pages

II. Causes of fluid and electrolyte imbalances: 50%–75% of clients with cancer have imbalances caused by alterations in intake or metabolism.

A. Cachexia: complex of biochemical abnormalities occurring as the result of cancer
  1. Causes: altered metabolism of all major nutrients
     a) Glucose metabolism higher than normal
     b) More anaerobic use of nutrients, leading to increased lactic acid production; lactic acidosis
     c) Nitrogen moves from body tissues into tumor; negative nitrogen balance
     d) Sodium retained, but concentrated in tumor; hyponatremia
  2. Signs and symptoms: affects entire body; anorexia, weight loss, wasting, muscle weakness, fluid and electrolyte imbalances, increased basal metabolic rate, and anemia

B. Malabsorption syndrome: inflammation, ulceration, and decreased secretions of GI tract; protein and fat absorption altered leading to fluid and electrolyte imbalances

C. Third-space fluid accumulation: common
  1. Causes
     a) Malignant tumors secrete fluids into body cavities; most common cause
     b) Edema due to blocked lymphatic or venous return coupled with protein seepage from capillaries
  2. Effects: increase in total body fluids, with actual intravascular fluid volume deficit (FVD); signs and symptoms of FVD

D. Altered hormonal regulation: abnormal (ectopic) hormones secreted by cancer cells not subject to normal feedback regulation; excess causes severe fluid and electrolyte imbalances

1. Antidiuretic hormone (ADH): lung (oat cell cancer), pancreas, Hodgkin's disease, and prostate; causes syndrome of inappropriate ADH (SIADH), hyponatremia, and hypomagnesemia
2. Parathyroid hormone (PTH): lung, leukemia, multiple myeloma, and breast; causes hypercalcemia and hypophosphatemia
3. Adrenocorticotropic hormone (ACTH): lung (both oat cell and non–oat cell); causes hypokalemia
4. Osteoclast activating factor (OAF): multiple myeloma and lymphoma; causes hypercalcemia
5. Prostaglandins: breast, kidney, and pancreas; causes hypercalcemia

E. Treatment-related effects: specific imbalances associated with hormonal treatment, chemotherapy, and radiation; causes may be direct (e.g., tumor lysis) or indirect (e.g., side effects such as nausea and vomiting)

III. Specific fluid and electrolyte imbalances

See text pages

A. Hypercalcemia: serum calcium greater than 5.5 mEq/L; found in 10%–20% of all cancer clients
   1. Cancers associated with hypercalcemia: solid tumors with bony metastases (e.g., breast [40%–50% of clients], lung, kidney, colon, ovarian, prostate), solid tumors without bony metastases (e.g., lung, head and neck, kidney, ovarian, prostate), and hematological malignancies (e.g., leukemia, lymphoma)
   2. Causes of hypercalcemia: increased release of calcium from bone
      a) Tumor related: tumor lysis of bone, tumor release of PTH, tumor release of vitamin-D-like substances (for relationship of vitamin D to calcium regulation, see Chapter 3, section IV,A,6,c), immune cell release of OAF
      b) Treatment related: treatment with androgens, estrogens, progestins, and antiestrogens (e.g., tamoxifen for breast cancer)
   3. Signs and symptoms: anorexia, nausea, vomiting, muscle weakness, depression, apathy, psychosis (see Chapter 3, section IV,C,2, for more details)

B. Hypocalcemia: serum calcium less than 4.5 mEq/L
   1. Cancers associated with hypocalcemia: leukemia, lymphoma, and multiple myeloma
   2. Causes of hypocalcemia: malnutrition (main cause) secondary to liver disease, malabsorption syndrome, rapid bone healing after successful treatment of bony lesions (hungry bone syndrome), magnesium depletion, and tumor lysis (results in increased free phosphates that bind available calcium and form calcium phosphate precipitate)
   3. Signs and symptoms: paresthesia, tetany, irritability, and anxiety (see Chapter 3, section IV,B,2, for more details)

C. Hyperuricemia: serum uric acid greater than 8.0 mg/dl; uric acid crystals in urine
   1. Cancers associated with hyperuricemia: leukemia, lymphomas, and multiple myeloma

2. Causes of hyperuricemia
   a) Breakdown of cells; rapid release of nucleic acid from tumor lysis due to aggressive chemotherapy or radiation treatment
   b) Overproduction of uric acid precursors; common in polycythemia vera and chronic granulocytic leukemia
3. Signs and symptoms: blood in urine (hematuria), flank pain, nausea, vomiting, and precipitation of uric acid in kidneys leading to nephropathy and irreversible renal failure (see Chapter 10, section III, for signs and symptoms of renal failure)

D. Hyponatremia: serum sodium less than 135 mEq/L; very common
  1. Cancers associated with hyponatremia: lung, pancreatic, multiple myeloma, head and neck, brain, colon, ovarian, and prostate, all usually associated with dehydration; lung, pancreatic, brain, ovarian, colon, sarcoma, leukemia, prostate, Hodgkin's disease, and lymphomas, all associated with SIADH (dilutional hyponatremia)
  2. Causes of hyponatremia
   a) Liver, thyroid, and adrenal insufficiencies; renal failure; congestive heart failure; excess loss of sodium
   b) SIADH related: Increased ADH production by posterior pituitary or tumor at another site destroys feedback regulation.
   c) Treatment related: high doses of cyclophosphamide; daunorubicin or cytosine therapy; vincristine (SIADH)
  3. Signs and symptoms (see Chapter 3, section II,B,2)

E. Hyperkalemia: serum potassium greater than 5.0 mEq/L
  1. Cancers associated with hyperkalemia: lung (oat cell), liver, Hodgkin's disease, lymphoma, and leukemia
  2. Causes of hyperkalemia
   a) Redistribution of potassium: Potassium moves from cells into vascular fluid during metabolic or lactic acidosis.
   b) Treatment related: Lysis of large number of cells during radiation or chemotherapy releases potassium.
   c) Additional causes: renal failure; hypoaldosteronism
  3. Signs and symptoms (see Chapter 3, section III,C,2)

F. Hypokalemia: serum potassium less than 3.5 mEq/L
  1. Cancers associated with hypokalemia: colon, multiple myeloma, Hodgkin's disease, pancreatic, stomach, thyroid, adrenal, and cancers that release ectopic ACTH
  2. Causes of hypokalemia
   a) Insufficient dietary intake due to nausea and vomiting; increased loss due to diarrhea or fistula drainage

b) Treatment related: renal tubule damage caused by antibiotic therapy (e.g., gentamicin, carbenicillin, and cephalothin) as well as radiation and chemotherapy (elevated enzymes from massive cell lysis damage renal tubules)

c) Excessive urinary excretion of potassium: potassium-wasting diuretics, hypercalcemia, hypomagnesemia, ectopic ACTH secretion, and diuretic phase of renal failure from other causes

3. Signs and symptoms (see Chapter 3, section III,B,2)

G. Hyperphosphatemia: serum phosphorus greater than 4.5 mg/dl; usually occurs with hyperkalemia and hyperuricemia
   1. Cancers associated with hyperphosphatemia: leukemia, lymphoma, and multiple myeloma
   2. Causes of hyperphosphatemia: tumor lysis syndrome releasing large amounts of phosphates and renal failure from precipitation of calcium phosphate in kidney (see this chapter, section III,B,2)
   3. Signs and symptoms: oliguria, azotemia, and tetany (see Chapter 3, section VI,C,2, for more details)

H. Hypophosphatemia: serum phosphorus less than 2.5 mg/dl
   1. Cancers associated with hypophosphatemia: leukemia, multiple myeloma, and cancers that release ectopic PTH (PTH regulates phosphorus resorption)
   2. Causes of hypophosphatemia: excess PTH, aggressive parenteral nutrition (phosphate moves into cells during glucose metabolism), malabsorption, sepsis causing respiratory acidosis, diuretic use, and high phosphate use by aggressively growing malignancies
   3. Signs and symptoms: muscle weakness, irritability, numbness, paresthesia, confusion, seizures, and coma (see Chapter 3, section VI,B,2, for more details)

I. Hypomagnesemia: serum magnesium less than 1.3 mEq/L
   1. Cancers associated with hypomagnesemia: lung (oat cell), ovarian, and testicular
   2. Causes of hypomagnesemia: magnesium loss through severe diarrhea or vomiting, magnesium wasting due to treatment with cisplatin, treatment with antibiotics toxic to kidney (e.g., gentamicin), excessive ADH secretion, and total parenteral nutrition without adequate magnesium supplementation
   3. Signs and symptoms (see Chapter 3, section V,B,2)

J. Lactic (metabolic) acidosis: arterial blood pH less than 7.35, HCO_3 less than 22 mEq/L
   1. Cancers associated with lactic acidosis: Hodgkin's disease, lymphoma, leukemia, lymphosarcoma, and lung (oat cell)
   2. Causes of lactic acidosis: Malignant cells use the anaerobic pathway to metabolize glucose, creating excess lactic acid as a by-product.
   3. Signs and symptoms: elevated serum lactic acid; signs of metabolic acidosis (see Chapter 4, section II,B)

See text pages

IV. Treatment and management

A. General considerations
1. The underlying malignancy must be taken into consideration in any treatment of fluid and electrolyte imbalances in clients who have cancer.
2. Treatment of the underlying malignancy by radiation or chemotherapy is often the cause of fluid and electrolyte imbalances.
3. Treating the fluid and electrolyte problems and/or discontinuing cancer treatment may reverse life-threatening imbalances, but treatment of the underlying problem is needed for long-term correction.
4. Treatment of chronic fluid and electrolyte imbalances, as well as malignancies, may require long-term central venous access.

B. Considerations in specific fluid and electrolyte imbalances
1. Hypercalcemia
   a) Promote renal excretion of calcium: IV normal saline and diuretics that block calcium resorption (e.g., furosemide); short-term
   b) Reduce blood levels of calcium: hemodialysis and peritoneal dialysis; short-term

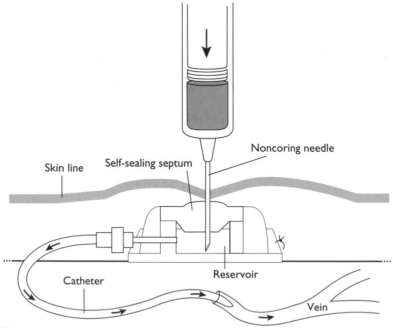

Figure 11–1
Implanted Device for Central Venous Access

     c) Inhibit bone resorption: medications such as mithramycin (antineoplastic antibiotic), calcitonin, and didronel; short-term

     d) Alter intake: reduce dietary calcium; short-term and long-term

     e) Remove sources of ectopic hormones and proteins: destroy tumors with radiation, chemotherapy, or surgical removal; long-term

     f) Reduce OAF: increase mobility; long-term

     g) Reduce absorption from gastrointestinal tract: phosphate salts and glucocorticoids; long-term

  2. Hyperuricemia

     a) Prevention: allopurinol before chemotherapy (inhibits uric acid formation), vigorous hydration, and alkalinization of urine

     b) Emergency: administer allopurinol, give fluids to improve hydration status, and increase urine pH to 7.0 or above; hemodialysis or peritoneal dialysis needed if renal damage has occurred

  3. Hyperphosphatemia: vigorous hydration and aluminum hydroxide to bind phosphate; hyperosmolar glucose and insulin (forces phosphate to move into cells); dialysis if renal failure is present

V. Nursing process

See text pages

A. Nursing assessment

  1. Assess for fluid and electrolyte imbalances; frequent reassessment is essential (see Nurse Alert, "Difficulties in Assessing Clients with Cancer").

  2. Assess for abnormal loss of electrolytes (e.g., severe diarrhea, vomiting, medications, anorexia).

  3. Assess laboratory test values.

B. Nursing diagnoses: normally collaborative

  1. Fluid volume deficit related to renal damage, decreased serum protein, and/or excessive sodium excretion

  2. Fluid volume excess related to increased levels of ADH

  3. High risk for injury related to bone demineralization

!　NURSE _ALERT_　!

Difficulties in Assessing Clients with Cancer

Fluid and electrolyte imbalances are difficult to assess in clients with cancer because the symptoms of imbalances (e.g., nausea, anorexia, muscle weakness) often mimic a client's response to chemotherapy or radiation. The nurse must make frequent re-assessments and take particular note of laboratory test values—especially after radiation, chemotherapy, surgery, or bone marrow transplants—to ascertain genuine fluid and electrolyte abnormalities.

4. Altered nutrition, less than body requirements, related to side effects of chemotherapy or radiation treatment
5. Altered urinary elimination related to hyperuricemia secondary to tumor lysis syndrome
6. Altered thought processes related to electrolyte imbalances

C. Nursing interventions
1. Monitor fluid and electrolyte status frequently via observations and laboratory tests.
2. Monitor urine output and composition.
3. Encourage small feedings of high-kcal, nonacidic foods and/or commercial supplements; administer tube feedings as needed.
4. Take safety precautions to prevent injury to brittle bones, especially if client's thought processes are altered.

1. A 40-year-old client in the terminal stage of Hodgkin's disease is receiving palliative care. The client has a fluid volume deficit and is cachexic. The nurse should assess the client for:

   a. Metabolic acidosis.
   b. Metabolic alkalosis.
   c. Respiratory acidosis.
   d. Respiratory alkalosis.

2. A 60-year-old client has a small-cell lung carcinoma. The client has 2+ edema affecting both feet and ankles and has a fasting blood glucose of 280 mg/dl. Based on these findings, the nurse should also assess the client for:

   a. Hyperphosphatemia.
   b. Hypernatremia.
   c. Hypokalemia.
   d. Hypomagnesemia.

3. A 5-year-old child with acute myelogenous leukemia has a white blood cell (WBC) count of 30,000/mm³. The nurse recognizes that this may cause false results in tests for:

   a. Sodium.
   b. Calcium.
   c. Chloride.
   d. Potassium.

4. An elderly client who has bone cancer is cachexic. The nurse recognizes that this client is at highest risk for a deficit of which of the following electrolytes?

   a. Calcium
   b. Magnesium
   c. Sodium
   d. Phosphorus

5. A 55-year-old client has colon cancer that has spread to the adjacent surface of the liver. Which of the following nursing diagnoses is most likely to apply to this client?

   a. Fluid volume excess, hypervolemia, related to increased permeability of intestinal mucosa

   b. Altered thought processes related to cerebral edema due to increased intracellular fluid

   c. Risk for impaired skin integrity related to circulatory impairment secondary to peripheral edema

   d. Fluid volume deficit, hypovolemia, related to third spacing of fluid in abdominal cavity

6. A female client has advanced breast cancer with metastases to the bone. Her serum calcium level is 16 mg/dl. Which of the following nursing diagnoses is most likely to be appropriate?

   a. Altered thought processes related to neurologic effects of hypercalcemia

   b. Diarrhea related to calcium-induced hypermotility of the bowel

   c. Fluid volume excess related to osmotic effect of excess calcium

   d. Pain related to muscle cramping due to neuromuscular excitability

7. A client has oat cell carcinoma of the lung and receives large doses of narcotics for pain control. The client has developed an intracellular fluid volume excess. The most likely etiology of this problem is:

   a. Excessive ADH secretion.
   b. Increased sodium excretion.
   c. Increased fluid intake due to thirst.
   d. Hyperactivity of the adrenal glands.

8. A 30-year-old client is scheduled to receive the first course of chemotherapy for acute myelogenous leukemia. The nurse should anticipate pretreatment orders for:

   a. Plicamycin (Mithracin).
   b. Vitamin C.
   c. Allopurinol (Zyloprim).
   d. Hydrochlorothiazide (HydroDIURIL).

9. A 47-year-old client has advanced pancreatic cancer. The client's food intake is poor. The client complains of discomfort from swollen ankles. Which of the following should the nursing care plan include?

   a. Offering several times a day snacks that are high in sodium
   b. Encouraging use of nonsteroidal anti-inflammatory drugs (NSAIDs) to manage pain
   c. Keeping the legs elevated as much as possible when out of bed
   d. Offering small amounts of high-carbohydrate fluids every hour

10. A 42-year-old woman takes tamoxifen (Nolvadex) on an outpatient basis to treat breast cancer. The nurse should teach this client to:

    a. Rest in bed or a chair as much as possible.
    b. Drink 3–4 liters of fluid daily—especially broths.
    c. Consume more dairy products.
    d. Eat foods that are low in residue.

11. A 25-year-old client with leukemia is being treated with chemotherapy. During the induction phase of the chemotherapy, a low phosphate diet is prescribed. The nurse should instruct the client to avoid:

    a. Fresh fruits.
    b. Red meats.
    c. Tea.
    d. Hard cheeses.

12. A 10-year-old child has acute lymphoblastic leukemia. During the induction phase of this client's chemotherapy, the nurse should observe the child carefully for:

    a. Rapid, deep respirations.
    b. Arrhythmias and postural hypotension.
    c. Flank pain and hematuria.
    d. Thirst and excessive urine output.

ANSWERS

1. **Correct answer is a.** The cachexia of cancer involves many biochemical abnormalities. Because glucose utilization is higher in cancer cells, anaerobic metabolism occurs. It results in accumulation of lactic acid, which produces metabolic acidosis.

   b. Anaerobic metabolism causes acid by-products to accumulate, thereby producing acidosis. Metabolic alkalosis usually occurs during periods of vomiting secondary to chemotherapy.
   c and d. Cachexia involves metabolic changes that lead to accumulation of acid wastes. Neither respiratory acidosis nor respiratory alkalosis is likely as a complication of cachexia.

2. **Correct answer is c.** Edema and hyperglycemia are signs of ectopic adrenocorticotropic hormone (ACTH) production, which is a potential complication of small-cell lung carcinomas. The increased circulating ACTH promotes renal potassium excretion, thereby producing hypokalemia.

   a. Hyperphosphatemia is an uncommon complication, which generally results from destruction of large numbers of cancer cells.
   b. Hypernatremia is most likely to occur if a cancer such as multiple myeloma causes renal damage.
   d. Hypomagnesemia occurs when cisplatin causes renal magnesium wasting due to its nephrotoxic effects.

3. **Correct answer is d.** The WBC count is elevated (normal for child = 4500–13,500/mm³). Large numbers of fragile leukocytes in a blood sample increase cell lysis. Potassium released from the damaged cells falsely elevates the potassium level in the specimen.

   a, b, and **c.** None of these electrolytes is affected by the presence of large numbers of WBCs.

4. **Correct answer is b.** Potassium and magnesium deficits are the most common imbalances associated with cachexia.

   a. Bone cancers increase the risk for hypercalcemia due to bone demineralization.

c. Poor oral intake may lead to fluid volume deficit. Fluid volume deficit due to decreased fluid intake is often associated with hypernatremia.

d. Phosphorus depletion is more often seen when nutritional status improves and formation of new tissue consumes phosphorus.

5. **Correct answer is d.** Invasive colon cancer involves the serous membranes of the peritoneum, producing effusion into the abdominal cavity. The high protein content of that effusion helps to prevent the fluid from being resorbed. Because the fluid is trapped outside the vascular space, hypovolemia results.

   a. Hypervolemia is unlikely. The absorptive capacity of the intestinal mucosa does not increase in cancer. Absorption may be decreased if there is partial or complete obstruction.

   b. Hypovolemia will develop due to peritoneal effusions. Serum electrolyte concentration increases in hypovolemia (hyperosmolality). Cerebral edema develops when serum is hypo-osmolar.

   c. Peripheral edema develops when hydrostatic pressure increases secondary to hypervolemia. This client is more likely to become hypovolemic.

6. **Correct answer is a.** Hypercalcemia produces reversible mental status changes such as confusion, disorientation, and memory loss.

   b. Calcium relaxes smooth muscle. This reduces gastrointestinal motility, resulting in constipation.

   c. Urinary calcium levels increase as a result of hypercalcemia. The high levels of calcium in the blood produce osmotic effects that result in polyuria. Fluid volume deficit ensues.

   d. Muscle cramping is associated with hypocalcemia. Increased calcium levels have a sedating effect at the myoneural junction, resulting in muscle weakness.

7. **Correct answer is a.** SIADH is a common complication of lung tumors. Narcotics also stimulate ADH release. ADH promotes resorption of water by the kidneys. Much of the excess water retained in SIADH moves into cells, causing intracellular fluid volume excess, or water intoxication.

   b. Water is drawn toward sodium by osmotic forces. If sodium excretion increases, water excretion will also increase.

   c. Clients who have cancer usually have reduced oral intake. Lung cancer does not stimulate increased thirst.

   d. Adrenal hyperactivity would increase aldosterone levels. Aldosterone causes fluid and sodium retention. Lung cancer, however, does not stimulate increased adrenal activity.

8. **Correct answer is c.** Because cancer cells have high growth rates, they contain more nucleic acids than normal cells do. Metabolism of the excess nucleic acids that are released when large numbers of cancer cells are destroyed elevates uric acid levels. Prophylactic treatment includes administration of allopurinol, which reduces uric acid production.

   a. Mithracin is used to treat hypercalcemia. It is an antineoplastic drug that would destroy cancer cells, adding to the hyperuricemia.

   b. Vitamin C acidifies urine. Uric acid is excreted more efficiently in alkaline urine.

   d. Thiazide diuretics such as Hydro-DIURIL are to be avoided because they compete with uric acid for excretion sites, thus elevating uric acid levels.

9. **Correct answer is c.** Clients with cancer frequently have low albumin levels. Poor intake, impaired liver synthesis, and alterations in metabolism contribute to decreased albumin. When albumin is low, plasma oncotic pressure is decreased. For that reason, clients with cancer are prone to develop dependent edema. Elevating the legs reduces hydrostatic pressure, thus decreasing the edema.

   a. Increased sodium would further increase the risk for edema in a client with low albumin levels.

   b. NSAIDs promote sodium and fluid retention, which would contribute to the risk for peripheral edema.

d. Increased carbohydrate would not help prevent edema. High-protein fluids would be a better choice, as they would help raise albumin levels.

10. **Correct answer is b.** Clients with breast cancer are at risk for hypercalcemia. Anti-estrogens, such as tamoxifen, increase the risk. To promote calcium excretion and prevent formation of renal stones, the client should drink 3–4 liters of fluid daily. Broth provides extra sodium, which facilitates renal calcium excretion.

    a. Mobility, especially weight bearing, helps to decrease osteoclastic activity, reducing calcium release from bones. Activity should be encouraged.
    c. Dairy products are high in calcium. Dietary calcium should be limited because hypercalcemia is likely.
    d. Hypercalcemia causes constipation. Dietary fiber should be encouraged to help prevent constipation.

11. **Correct answer is d.** Hard cheeses, milk-based desserts, dried fruits, nuts, and whole-grain cereals are high in phosphates and should be avoided.

    a. Dried fruits are contraindicated, but fresh fruits are permitted.
    b. Some specialty meats, such as kidneys, would be limited, but most meats are permitted in a low-phosphate diet.
    c. Tea is not high in phosphates and would not be contraindicated.

12. **Correct answer is c.** Rapid destruction of large numbers of cells releases excess uric acid. Flank pain and hematuria are signs of hyperuricemia. Uric acid precipitates in the kidneys and may lead to renal failure.

    a. This would indicate respiratory compensation for metabolic acidosis. Elevations of electrolytes and uric acid occur with tumor lysis syndrome. Acidosis is associated with cachexia.
    b. These are associated with hypokalemia. Tumor lysis syndrome includes hyperkalemia, because cell destruction releases large amounts of potassium.
    d. These are associated with hypercalcemia. Calcium levels fall in tumor lysis syndrome because phosphates released from the destroyed cancer cells form calcium phosphate, lowering the serum level.

12

Diabetic Ketoacidosis and Hyperosmolar Coma

NURSING HIGHLIGHTS

1. Diabetic ketoacidosis and hyperglycemic hyperosmolar nonketotic coma differ in age of onset, speed of onset, and impact on acid-base balance, although both are related to ineffective metabolism of glucose.
2. Management of both diabetic ketoacidosis and hyperglycemic hyperosmolar nonketotic coma is similar and includes rehydration, insulin administration, and restoration of electrolyte balance.
3. While a client is receiving IV fluids and insulin, the nurse must monitor for signs of hypoglycemia (insulin reaction), which include headache, pallor, sweating, anxiety, tachycardia, blurred vision, and slurred speech.

GLOSSARY

hyperglycemia—elevated blood glucose level
insulin-dependent diabetes mellitus (IDDM, type I diabetes)—inability of the body to use glucose due to a severe or complete failure to secrete insulin; normally appears before age 30; requires outside source of insulin

non-insulin-dependent diabetes mellitus (NIDDM, type II diabetes)— inability of the body to use glucose due to resistance or decreased tissue response to insulin; normally appears after age 40; insulin level may be normal, elevated, or depressed; usually responds to diet and weight control

ENHANCED OUTLINE

See text pages

I. Pathophysiology and etiology: Diabetes mellitus is a complex metabolic disorder involving an absolute or relative lack of insulin or decreased tissue response to insulin that causes the body to fail to metabolize glucose and produces severe hyperglycemia.

A. Diabetic ketoacidosis (DKA): associated with IDDM; may be first sign of undiagnosed diabetes
   1. Role of insulin
      a) Insulin is secreted by pancreatic beta cells.
      b) In absence of insulin, cells are impermeable to glucose; blood glucose levels rise (hyperglycemia).
      c) In absence of insulin, fats and proteins are broken down to provide body with energy.
      d) By-products of fat and protein catabolism are ketoacids, or ketones, such as B-hydroxybutyrate and acetoacetate (acetone).
   2. Development of DKA
      a) Liver fails to oxidize ketones.
      b) Ketone concentration in blood rises.
      c) Body becomes acidotic.
   3. Causes of DKA
      a) Insulin deficiency: undiagnosed IDDM; failure to take prescribed insulin, failure of insulin pump
      b) Physiologic stress: trauma, pancreatitis, infection, major surgery, gastroenteritis, dehydration, myocardial infarction, and pregnancy
      c) Additional causes: psychologic or emotional stress

B. Hyperglycemic hyperosmolar nonketotic (HHNK) coma: associated with NIDDM
   1. Development of HHNK coma: more gradual than DKA
      a) Insulin secretion may be normal, elevated, or depressed.
      b) Peripheral cells become refractory to insulin; blood glucose levels rise (hyperglycemia).
      c) Frequently, clients who develop HHNK coma are obese.
      d) Onset is gradual (days, weeks).

    2. Causes of HHNK coma

        a) Physiologic stress: renal impairment, cardiovascular disease, infection, trauma, burns, and surgery

        b) Drug treatment: mannitol, steroids, thiazide diuretics, phenytoin, and chlorpromazine

        c) Peritoneal dialysis

        d) Rapid initiation of total parenteral nutrition (TPN) or tube feeding (see Chapter 5, section V,D)

C. Hypoglycemia and other causes of coma

    1. Hypoglycemia (low blood glucose)

        a) Symptoms: headache, pallor, sweating, anxiety, tachycardia, hunger, weakness, dizziness, visual and speech disturbances, and convulsions

        b) Test for hypoglycemia: IV 50% glucose or intramuscular glucagon to relieve symptoms (see Nurse Alert, "Eliminating Hypoglycemia as a Possible Cause of Coma").

    2. Other conditions with symptoms that resemble DKA or HHNK coma: stroke, uremia, drug intoxication, and alcoholic ketoacidosis

II. Signs and symptoms

See text pages
_____

A. Diabetic ketoacidosis

    1. Vital signs: slightly elevated or normal temperature, rapid pulse, postural hypotension (reduced blood pressure if severe), weight loss, and Kussmaul breathing (compensation for acidosis)

    2. Laboratory signs

        a) Blood glucose: 300–4000 mg/dl; above 180 mg/dl, glucose appears in urine (glycosuria)

        b) pH: <7.3

        c) Serum bicarbonate (HCO_3): <14 mEq/L (compensation for high levels of anionic ketones)

        d) Serum osmolality: elevated (normal is 280–295 mOsm/kg)

      e) Hemoglobin and hematocrit: elevated due to fluid volume deficit (FVD)

      f) Urine specific gravity: elevated due to glycosuria and ketonuria (ketones in urine)

3. Hyperglycemia: fatigue, muscle weakness, blurred vision, oliguria or anuria (severe, late symptom), and depressed level of consciousness

4. FVD: polyuria due to osmotic diuresis, extreme thirst, weakness, fatigue, nausea, vomiting, poor skin and tongue turgor, and weight loss

5. Ketoacidosis: abdominal pain (preceded by anorexia, nausea, vomiting), bright red skin and mucous membranes, Kussmaul breathing, and fruity smell on breath (acetone expired to reduce ketone load)

6. Electrolyte imbalances

      a) Potassium: total body deficit—elevated in serum and low in cells; affected by cellular breakdown, potassium-losing effects of aldosterone, and potassium and fluid loss due to osmotic diuresis, anorexia, and vomiting

      b) Sodium: usually lowered; lost during osmotic diuresis, vomiting, and dehydration; high within potassium-depleted cells

      c) Phosphorus: usually lowered; same causes as potassium

B. HHNK coma

1. Vital signs: slightly elevated or normal temperature, rapid pulse, postural hypotension (reduced blood pressure if severe), and weight loss

2. FVD: polyuria and extreme thirst as well as weakness and standard signs of FVD

3. Laboratory signs:

      a) Blood glucose: 400–4800 mg/dl (higher than DKA)

      b) pH: normal or slightly decreased

      c) HCO_3: normal or slightly lowered (no buildup of ketones)

      d) Serum osmolality: >350 mOsm/kg

      e) Blood urea nitrogen (BUN): elevated, 60–90 mg/dl

      f) Serum creatinine: often elevated; related to renal impairment

4. Hyperglycemia: more pronounced than with DKA (see section II,A,3 of this chapter)

5. FVD: more pronounced than with DKA (see section II,A,4 of this chapter)

6. Electrolyte imbalances (see section II,A,6 of this chapter)

III. Treatment and management

See text pages
_____

A. Fluid replacement: essential to prevent renal and cardiovascular damage

1. Initial infusion of iso-osmolar saline (0.9% NaCl), 1–3 liters

2. Continued infusion with half-strength saline (0.45% NaCl)

3. After plasma glucose measures 250–300 mg/dl, glucose added to prevent hypoglycemia

B. Insulin administration: Goal is to give enough regular (rapid-acting) insulin to correct problem without driving client into hypoglycemia.
   1. IV administration is best; second choice is either intramuscular or subcutaneous administration.
   2. Large doses are no better than small doses for correcting DKA; small doses lower blood glucose more smoothly.
   3. Clients with HHNK coma may need larger doses than clients with DKA.
   4. Use of controlled-rate infusion pump or volume-controlled administration set regulates delivery to prevent hypoglycemia or cerebral edema (from rapid change in serum osmolality).

C. Electrolyte replacement
   1. Potassium
      a) Usually added to 0.45% NaCl after initial IV infusion of iso-osmolar NaCl and establishment of improved urine output
      b) Risk of added potassium's causing hyperkalemia; frequent monitoring of serum level and electrocardiogram needed
   2. Phosphorus: lost during osmotic diuresis of DKA and HHNK coma; replacement controversial

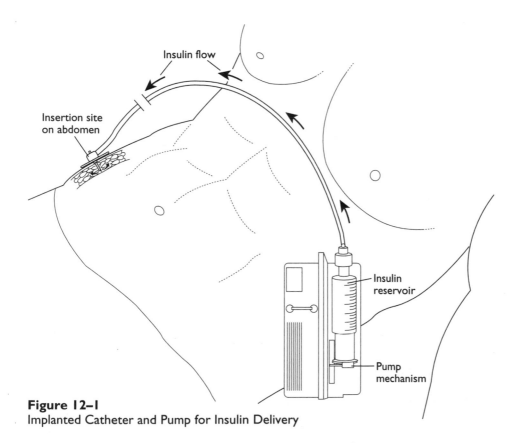

Figure 12–1
Implanted Catheter and Pump for Insulin Delivery

        a) Excess replacement causes hyperphosphatemia and hypocalcemia.

        b) Kidney must be functioning well before replacement is started.

    3. Sodium: replaced through administration of iso-osmolar and hypo-osmolar saline

    4. Bicarbonate: lost to compensate for buildup of ketones (anions) with DKA; replacement controversial

        a) Bicarbonate is given only when pH falls below 7.1.

        b) Too rapid infusion causes acid-base imbalances and hypokalemia.

See text pages

IV. Nursing process

A. Nursing assessment

    1. Obtain client's history, with emphasis on signs of fluid loss and related health problems.

    2. Assess vital signs, with emphasis on signs suggesting FVD (e.g., rapid pulse, postural hypotension, weight loss).

    3. Assess respiration for compensatory (Kussmaul) breathing.

    4. Assess laboratory test results for indications of hyperglycemia, FVD, and DKA (e.g., high blood glucose, elevated hematocrit, and decreased pH and HCO_3, respectively).

    5. Assess urine for specific gravity, glycosuria, ketonuria, and excessive volume.

B. Nursing diagnoses

    1. Fluid volume deficit related to hyperglycemia and polyuria

    2. Altered nutrition, less than body requirements, related to failure to effectively metabolize glucose

    3. Altered renal, cardiovascular, and/or peripheral tissue perfusion related to fluid volume deficit

    4. Alteration in acid-base balance related to buildup of ketones in bloodstream

    5. Alteration in electrolyte balance (e.g., potassium, phosphorus) related to fluid volume deficit

    6. High risk for uncontrolled diabetes related to excessive physical or psychologic stress or insufficient management

    7. High risk for fluid volume excess related to excess administration of IV fluids

    8. High risk for hypoglycemia related to IV administration of insulin

C. Nursing interventions

    1. Monitor vital signs for changes in hydration status.

    2. Monitor changes in serum osmolality from laboratory reports.

    3. Monitor blood glucose levels frequently.

4. Monitor for indications of acid-base imbalance and response to therapy for DKA.
5. Monitor for indications of electrolyte imbalances and changes in electrolyte status in response to replacement therapy.
6. Administer IV fluids and insulin as directed by physician.
7. Monitor for signs of hypoglycemia in reaction to insulin administration.
8. Educate client on how to check his or her own blood glucose and urine glucose levels.
9. Assess client's understanding of insulin administration: technique as well as relationship to diet, exercise, illness, and stress; reeducate as indicated.

1. A 15-year-old client is admitted with a history of nausea and vomiting followed by abdominal pain. Blood test results include sodium (Na) = 125 mEq/L, chloride (Cl) = 85 mEq/L, pH = 7.29, HCO_3 = 12 mEq/L, $PaCO_2$ = 28 mm Hg, and glucose = 1624 mg/dl. Which of the following nursing interpretations of those assessments is most accurate?

   a. The client has hypochloremic alkalosis with respiratory compensation.
   b. The client has uncompensated respiratory acidosis.
   c. The client has a metabolic acidosis (diabetic ketoacidosis [DKA]) with respiratory compensation.
   d. The client has respiratory acidosis with metabolic compensation.

2. A middle-aged person is found unconscious and wearing a Medic Alert ID indicating diabetes. To distinguish between hypoglycemia and hyperglycemia, which of the following would be appropriate to do?

   a. Administer 50 ml of 50% glucose IV.
   b. Give 5 units of regular insulin IV.
   c. Give 500 ml of normal saline IV.
   d. Place 1 oz of sugar under the tongue.

3. A 69-year-old client with non-insulin-dependent diabetes mellitus (NIDDM) has not taken the prescribed glyburide (Micronase) for a week. The client has nausea, dizziness, blurred vision, and fatigue. Blood glucose is 625 mg/dl. Which nursing diagnosis is most likely to apply to this client?

   a. Altered sodium balance (hypernatremia) related to increased aldosterone secretion
   b. Fluid volume deficit related to the osmotic effects of glycosuria
   c. Altered calcium balance (hypercalcemia) related to increased release of calcium from bones
   d. Fluid volume excess related to shifting of fluid from the intracellular to the intravascular space

4. A 70-year-old client with hyperglycemic hyperosmolar nonketotic (HHNK) coma related to NIDDM is being treated with IV normal saline and insulin. Blood glucose on admission was 3750 mg/dl. If blood glucose falls too rapidly, the nurse would observe signs of:

   a. Ketosis.
   b. Cerebral edema.
   c. Hyperkalemia.
   d. Respiratory alkalosis.

5. A 35-year-old client with IDDM has diabetic ketoacidosis. IV fluids are started. Which of the following fluids should the nurse anticipate an order to hang?

   a. D_5W with insulin
   b. Half-strength saline with potassium
   c. Ringer's solution
   d. Normal saline

6. A 50-year-old client was admitted with HHNK coma. On admission, the client was hypotensive and oliguric. The client has received 2 liters of normal saline and 40 units of regular insulin IV over the past 2 hours. The next order calls for 1 liter of half-strength saline with 40 mEq of potassium chloride. The nurse would not administer that solution if:

   a. Serum potassium is 3.8 mEq/L.
   b. Urine output is 20 ml in 1 hour.
   c. Serum sodium is 138 mEq/L.
   d. Urine specific gravity is 1.045.

7. A client is receiving an IV of 5% dextrose in half-strength saline with potassium to treat DKA. Blood glucose is now 450 mg/dl. To help correct the hypophosphatemia that occurs with osmotic diuresis, which of the following should the client be offered?

   a. Chicken broth
   b. Tomato juice
   c. Pineapple juice
   d. Skim milk

8. A 12-year-old child with IDDM takes 25 units of isophane insulin suspension (Humulin N) daily. The child has an upper respiratory infection and has not been eating well. The child's parent asks about giving the prescribed insulin. The nurse should tell the parent to:

   a. Give half the insulin and encourage the child to drink high-glucose juices.
   b. Withhold the insulin if the child's urine tests positive for ketones.
   c. Give the insulin only if the child eats breakfast.
   d. Give the child 25 units of insulin and test the child's blood glucose every 4 hours.

9. A 22-year-old client with IDDM has an arthroscopy to repair a torn meniscus in the short procedure unit. In addition to the client's being given the usual discharge instructions, which of the following symptoms should this client be told to report to the physician?

   a. Excessive urine output
   b. Insomnia
   c. Edema of the feet and ankles
   d. Tinnitus

10. A 70-year-old client with NIDDM is being treated for HHNK coma. The client receives 2 liters of normal saline IV over a 2-hour period initially. For which complication should the nurse monitor the client during that time?

   a. Circulatory overload
   b. Hypochloremia
   c. Hyperkalemia
   d. Metabolic alkalosis

11. A client has had NIDDM for 10 years and has developed renal insufficiency. Because the client is at risk for HHNK coma, the nurse should observe for:

   a. Fruity breath odor.
   b. Deep, rapid respirations.
   c. Postural hypotension.
   d. Profuse sweating.

12. A client is unconscious when admitted for treatment of DKA. ABGs on admission are pH = 7.04, HCO_3 = 8 mEq/L, and $PaCO_2$ = 22 mm Hg. Respirations are deep and respiratory rate is 34. For which indication of worsening condition should the nurse monitor this client?

   a. Carpal spasms when BP is taken
   b. Frequent muscle twitching
   c. Labored, shallow breathing
   d. Cherry-red oral mucous membranes

ANSWERS

1. Correct answer is c. Although the pH is low, the high anion gap (AG—the difference between the Na level and the combined levels of HCO_3 [bicarbonate] and Cl) indicates more-severe metabolic acidosis than the pH shows. Using the formula $AG = Na - (HCO_3 + Cl)$, the AG is determined to measure 28 mEq/L (125 – [12 + 85]). Normal AG is less than 16 mEq/L. DKA is a high-AG acidosis. The history of abdominal pain following nausea and vomiting is consistent with DKA. The low $PaCO_2$ (partial pressure of carbon dioxide [CO_2] in arterial blood) indicates respiratory compensation.

   a. The client does have hypochloremia, but the pH of 7.29 indicates a primary acidosis.
   b and **d.** The low $PaCO_2$ would produce respiratory alkalosis, so the acidosis is not of respiratory origin.

2. Correct answer is a. This amount of 50% glucose IV would rapidly correct hypoglycemia. If hyperglycemia is the problem, glucose would not seriously worsen it.

   b. Insulin would dangerously worsen the client's condition if the client is hypoglycemic.
   c. Fluid would not correct hypoglycemia. This amount of fluid is not enough to improve dehydration due to hyperglycemia that is severe enough to cause coma.
   d. Sublingual absorption is not as reliable as IV. This amount of sugar may not be enough to improve the client's condition.

3. Correct answer is b. When blood glucose exceeds the renal threshold of 180 mg/dl, glucose is excreted in urine. Increased urine osmolality results in increased fluid and electrolyte losses, leaving the client dehydrated.

a. Increased aldosterone secretion is not a response to hyperglycemia. Sodium shifts into cells as potassium shifts out, and hyponatremia occurs.
c. Hyperglycemia does not increase release of calcium from bones. Hypocalcemia sometimes occurs due to increased urinary excretion of calcium.
d. Hyperglycemia shifts fluid from the intracellular to the intravascular space. Glycosuria causes excretion of that fluid in urine, resulting in fluid volume deficit.

4. Correct answer is b. Glucose enters brain cells without the mediation of insulin. If blood glucose is reduced rapidly, the osmotic gradient pulls fluid into brain cells, causing cerebral edema.

a. Clients with NIDDM generally do not develop ketosis. In any case, insulin would reduce the risk for ketosis by moving glucose into cells.
c. Insulin drives potassium back into cells, leaving the client hypokalemic.
d. Respiratory alkalosis occurs with hyperventilation. Fluids and insulin reduce the risk of acidosis, thereby reducing compensatory hyperventilation.

5. Correct answer is d. Isotonic saline is usually the first fluid used to rehydrate a client with DKA.

a. Dextrose solutions are not initiated until blood glucose has been reduced to 250–300 mg/dl.
b. Potassium is not replaced until 2–3 liters of IV fluid have been administered and adequate urinary output is achieved. If potassium is replaced while renal function is inadequate, hyperkalemia could occur.
c. The high chloride content in Ringer's solution can increase acidosis. If a Ringer's

solution were given, it would most likely be lactated Ringer's, which would help reduce the metabolic acidosis.

6. Correct answer is b. Continued low urine output may indicate renal failure due to prolonged dehydration. Potassium is not administered until adequate renal function has been established.

a. Potassium may be normal initially, but it will fall as urine output rises and plasma volume expands and as potassium shifts into cells with insulin and glucose. Potassium is given to prevent a precipitous drop in potassium.
c. This is a normal sodium level. As potassium shifts into cells, sodium shifts into the serum, tending to maintain normal sodium levels.
d. Increased urine specific gravity occurs with fluid volume deficit and glycosuria. Heavy glycosuria invalidates urine specific gravity results.

7. Correct answer is d. Skim milk is a good source of phosphorus.

a. Chicken broth is high in sodium but low in phosphorus.
b. Tomato juice is a good source of sodium and potassium, but is low in phosphorus.
c. Pineapple juice is a good source of potassium, but is low in phosphorus.

8. Correct answer is d. The child needs the regular dose of insulin and may need extra insulin to prevent hyperglycemia and DKA due to the illness.

a. The child is at greater risk for hyperglycemia than hypoglycemia. Insulin doses should not be altered without physician's orders.
b. Testing urine for ketones is a good idea. However, ketonuria indicates the need for more insulin, not less.
c. The child needs to receive insulin even if no food is eaten. If the child cannot keep food down, the physician should be consulted.

9. **Correct answer is a.** Physiologic stresses in trauma and surgery increase the risk for hyperglycemia and DKA. Polyuria is an early sign of hyperglycemia and should be reported.

b. Somnolence, not insomnia, is associated with hyperglycemia.
c. This is a sign of hypervolemia. Hyperglycemia causes hypovolemia.
d. Blurred vision is a sign of DKA. Tinnitus is not associated with DKA.

10. **Correct answer is a.** IV fluids rapidly correct the extracellular fluid deficit in HHNK coma. Fluid moves into cells more slowly. During the initial rapid administration of normal saline, hypervolemia can occur.

b. Normal saline contains more chloride than plasma. Chloride levels remain normal in HHNK coma unless vomiting has occurred. Hyperchloremia is more likely.
c. Hyperkalemia may be present initially, but potassium levels fall during treatment and hypokalemia may occur.
d. Normal saline is not an alkaline solution, so metabolic alkalosis is not a complication of therapy. If hyperchloremia occurs, metabolic acidosis would be likely.

11. **Correct answer is c.** Clients with HHNK coma develop profound fluid volume deficit.

Postural hypotension is an early sign and would be helpful in recognizing a developing HHNK coma.

a and **b.** These are signs of ketosis, which does not occur in HHNK coma. They would be present in a client with DKA.
d. This is a sign of hypoglycemia. It would not occur in HHNK coma.

12. **Correct answer is c.** A shift to shallow, gasping breaths may indicate either a drop in pH below 7.0 or impaired perfusion of the respiratory center due to circulatory collapse. Either would reflect serious worsening of the client's condition.

a. Carpopedal spasms are associated with metabolic alkalosis and hypocalcemia. Because this client is not vomiting, metabolic alkalosis is not likely. DKA does not affect serum calcium levels.
b. Muscle twitching is associated with respiratory acidosis. Because respirations are deep and rapid, this client is unlikely to develop respiratory acidosis. The low $PaCO_2$ is compensatory.
d. This indicates peripheral vasodilation, which occurs in response to ketosis. This is an expected finding in DKA and does not indicate a worsening of the condition.

Fluids and Electrolytes Comprehensive Review Questions

1. Which of the following associated body fluid changes is a client admitted for protein-kcal malnutrition most likely to have?
   a. Peripheral edema
   b. Cerebral edema
   c. Hyperkalemia
   d. Hypokalemia

2. To ensure the accuracy of weights that are taken to monitor fluid volume changes, a client's weight should be obtained:
   a. In the morning, after the client uses the bathroom.
   b. Immediately upon arising, before the client ambulates.
   c. At bedtime, before any bedtime snack is consumed.
   d. Anytime during the day that dependent edema is observed.

3. A 72-year-old client has moderate fluid volume deficit. In addition to fluid replacement, the nursing care plan for this client should include:
   a. Sodium restriction.
   b. Bed rest until vital signs are normal.
   c. Daily bathing with an antimicrobial soap.
   d. Frequent mouth care.

4. A client has mild congestive heart failure. To help prevent extracellular fluid excess, the nurse should teach the client to:
   a. Drink only electrolyte-free fluids.
   b. Sleep with the head of the bed elevated.
   c. Lie down to rest several times a day.
   d. Increase dietary calcium intake.

5. The nurse should teach the client for whom a potassium supplement is prescribed to:
   a. Take the medication 1 hour before or 2 hours after eating.
   b. Drink liquid supplement through a straw to avoid staining the teeth.
   c. Take slow-release tablets with 1 or 2 sips of water.
   d. Wait until effervescent preparations stop fizzing before drinking them.

6. A client with a 20-year history of alcoholism is admitted to the hospital for detoxification prior to entering a rehabilitation program. During the period of alcohol withdrawal, it is especially important to monitor this client's serum levels of:
   a. Sodium.
   b. Potassium.
   c. Chloride.
   d. Magnesium.

7. A client's arterial blood gas (ABG) results are pH = 7.36, $PaCO_2$ = 27 mm Hg, HCO_3 = 18 mEq/L, and BE (base excess) = −4.8 mEq/L. The nurse recognizes that this client has:
   a. Uncompensated metabolic acidosis.
   b. Compensated metabolic acidosis.
   c. Uncompensated respiratory acidosis.
   d. Compensated respiratory acidosis.

8. A client presents at a walk-in clinic in a hysterical state. The client complains of blurred vision, tinnitus, and palpitations. The client has severe hand tremors and is diaphoretic. Immediate treatment for this client should include:
   a. Administering low-flow oxygen by nasal cannula.
   b. Restraining the client to prevent self-injury.
   c. Having the client breathe into a paper bag.
   d. Having the client drink an electrolyte replacement solution.

9. A client is receiving dextran 70 to treat hypovolemic shock. For which complication of such therapy should the nurse closely monitor this client?

   a. Hyperkalemia
   b. Bleeding
   c. Metabolic alkalosis
   d. Dehydration

10. Total parenteral nutrition is ordered to treat a client's malnutrition. To monitor the client for the development of nutritional recovery syndrome, the nurse should periodically assess for:

    a. Decreased grip strength.
    b. Hyperactive deep-tendon reflexes.
    c. Carpal spasms.
    d. Hypoactive bowel sounds.

11. A 3-year-old has a fluid volume deficit due to diarrhea. Urine output is low and skin turgor is poor, but the child is alert. The preferred method to rehydrate this client would be:

    a. Room-temperature water PO.
    b. IV normal saline.
    c. Electrolyte and glucose solution PO.
    d. IV 5% dextrose in water.

12. The nurse has determined that an 85-year-old client is at risk for acidosis due to age-related changes. To prevent acidosis, the nurse should teach the client to:

    a. Reduce intake of acidic juices.
    b. Perform breathing exercises with prolonged expiration.
    c. Increase intake of foods that are high in potassium.
    d. Raise the head of the bed on blocks that are 6–8 inches.

13. A client is hospitalized after an automobile accident. On admission, the vital signs were blood pressure (BP) = 128/80, pulse (P) = 100, respirations (R) = 24, and temperature (T) = 98.6°. Which of the following

assessments 12 hours after the accident suggests a complication and should be reported to the physician?

   a. T = 99°
   b. BP = 118/80
   c. P = 106
   d. R = 30

14. A client is comatose following a basal skull fracture. The urine output is 200–300 ml/hour. Urine specific gravity is 1.002. Based on those observations, which of the following nursing diagnoses is appropriate at this time?

    a. Fluid volume excess related to release of excessive antidiuretic hormone (ADH)
    b. Risk for altered sodium balance (hypernatremia) related to reduced pituitary secretion of ADH
    c. Risk for altered potassium balance (hyperkalemia) related to deficient aldosterone release
    d. Hypothermia related to abnormalities in hypothalamic function

15. A client who takes cortisone for severe arthritis is admitted with adynamic ileus and hypovolemia. Which of the following test results would help identify the cause of the problem?

    a. Urine osmolality
    b. Serum osmolality
    c. Arterial blood gases
    d. Serum potassium

16. A 50-year-old client with alcoholism has acute pancreatitis. Vomiting and diarrhea have subsided because the client is receiving nothing by mouth and the nasogastric tube is clamped. IV fluids have maintained the urine output at 50 ml/hour. The client reports adequate pain control with meperidine (Demerol) every 4 hours. There is ascites, and chest x-ray shows left pleural effusion. For which acid-base imbalance should the nurse monitor the client at this time?

a. Respiratory acidosis
b. Respiratory alkalosis
c. Metabolic acidosis
d. Metabolic alkalosis

17. A 70-year-old client with congestive heart failure is being treated with digoxin and furosemide (Lasix). The nurse should teach the client to increase intake of:

a. Fruits.
b. Poultry.
c. Dairy products.
d. Breads.

18. A client has chronic obstructive pulmonary disease. The nurse notes that the client has a barrel chest and dyspnea on exertion. The client's expirations are prolonged. Which ABG result would indicate the presence of the acid-base imbalance for which the client is at greatest risk?

a. pH = 7.28
b. $PaCO_2$ = 32
c. HCO_3 = 24 mEq/L
d. BE = –2 mEq/L

19. A client with acute renal failure is being treated with peritoneal dialysis. The client receives 4 exchanges daily. On the third day of peritoneal dialysis, the client's serum potassium is 2.6 mEq/L. The nurse should anticipate an order to:

a. Increase the client's dietary potassium.
b. Administer an oral potassium supplement.
c. Administer an IV potassium supplement.
d. Add potassium to the dialysate for the next exchange.

20. A client has renal insufficiency due to hypertensive nephropathy. Which type of medication should the client be instructed to avoid using?

a. Nonsteroidal anti-inflammatory drugs (NSAIDs)
b. Adrenergic decongestants

c. Loop diuretics
d. Multiple vitamins containing iron

21. A 25-year-old client has a renal adenocarcinoma that is secreting parathyroid hormone (PTH). The nurse recognizes that this client is at risk for:

a. Metabolic acidosis.
b. Hypercalcemia.
c. Hypokalemia.
d. Syndrome of inappropriate ADH.

22. A female client is receiving high-dose IV cyclophosphamide (Cytoxan) to treat ovarian cancer. The nurse should instruct her to call the physician if which of the following occurs in the first 24 hours?

a. Swelling of the hands or feet
b. Headache
c. Excessive thirst
d. Leg cramps

23. A 30-year-old client with insulin-dependent diabetes mellitus has diabetic ketoacidosis. On admission, blood pH was 7.14 and blood glucose was 950 mg/dl. On the first day, the client received 5 liters of fluid and 80 units of regular insulin. Blood pH is now 7.3, and blood glucose is 250 mg/dl. This client must be monitored for:

a. Flushed, dry skin.
b. Kussmaul breathing.
c. Pallor and diaphoresis.
d. Diarrhea.

24. A client is admitted with hyperglycemic hyperosmolar nonketotic (HHNK) coma. The client is conscious but drowsy. To prevent the complications of HHNK coma, the nursing care plan should include:

a. Keeping the client in high Fowler's position.
b. Avoiding oral fluid intake.
c. Reducing carbohydrate and increasing fat in the diet.
d. Encouraging the client to exercise the legs frequently.

1. Correct answer is a. A diet deficient in protein leads to reduced serum protein. This reduces colloid osmotic (oncotic) pressure, which allows water to move out of the vascular space and into the interstitial space and produces peripheral edema.

b. Cerebral edema is most often a result of excessive intake of water without electrolytes. Free water shifts into cells—including brain cells—to equalize the osmolality of all fluid compartments.
c and d. Changes in serum potassium levels are not directly associated with protein-kcal malnutrition.

2. Correct answer is a. To ensure accuracy, the weight should be obtained in the morning. Both bladder and stomach should be empty, so the weight should be obtained after voiding and before eating or drinking.

b. Ambulation does not significantly affect weight.
c and d. Weights obtained during or at the end of the day are altered by eating, drinking, and diurnal variations.

3. Correct answer is d. Mucous membranes are often dry in fluid volume deficit. Frequent mouth care provides comfort and prevents damage to the mucosa.

a. Sodium restriction is not indicated in fluid volume deficit.
b. Bed rest is not necessary. Safety precautions, such as assistance while ambulating and slow position changes, may be indicated.
c. In fluid volume deficit, often the skin is dry. Antimicrobial soap would further dry the skin, which would be especially undesirable in an elderly client whose skin is already fragile. If daily bathing is important for hygiene, a mild soap or alternative cleaning agent should be used.

4. Correct answer is c. Lying down permits resorption of extracellular fluid and promotes diuresis.

a. Fluids high in sodium should be avoided, but other electrolytes are not contraindicated. Excessive intake of sodium-free fluids could cause water intoxication.
b. This position helps to relieve the dyspnea and orthopnea that result from pulmonary edema. It does not alter fluid retention.
d. Dietary sources of calcium include dairy products, which may add to sodium intake and exacerbate any edema that is present. In any case, calcium does not reduce fluid retention.

5. Correct answer is d. Potassium preparations should not be taken until they have dissolved completely. Effervescent products are completely dissolved when they stop fizzing.

a. This would be appropriate if the medication were to be taken on an empty stomach. Potassium should be taken with food to reduce gastrointestinal irritation.
b. Potassium does not stain teeth. This instruction is appropriate for liquid iron supplements.
c. Slow-release potassium tablets should be taken with a full glass of water to help them dissolve.

6. Correct answer is d. In the United States, chronic alcoholism is the most common cause of hypomagnesemia. Low serum magnesium levels may aggravate alcohol withdrawal symptoms.

a, b, and **c.** Although a chronic alcoholic may suffer from imbalances of any electrolyte due to altered nutritional status, none of these electrolytes is as commonly altered as magnesium.

7. Correct answer is b. Because the $PaCO_2$ (partial pressure of carbon dioxide [CO_2] in arterial blood) and HCO_3 (bicarbonate) levels are abnormal, an acid-base imbalance exists even though the pH is within normal limits. The pH is below 7.4, so the imbalance is acidotic. It is compensated because the pH is within the normal range (7.35–7.45). The HCO_3 is below normal, which is consistent with acidosis. Bicarbonate is regulated by the kidneys, so this is a metabolic acidosis. The lungs are compensating by reducing the carbon dioxide level ($PaCO_2$).

a and **c.** Because the pH is within the normal range, the imbalance must be compensated.
d. The respiratory component of the ABG results—$PaCO_2$—has shifted in the direction of increased alkalinity. Because that is in the opposite direction from the pH, the imbalance must be compensatory.

8. **Correct answer is c.** Hysteria is a common cause of respiratory alkalosis, and this client's symptoms are consistent with respiratory alkalosis. Breathing into a paper bag allows the client to rebreathe his or her own exhaled carbon dioxide to raise the $PaCO_2$.

a. Administering oxygen would raise the PaO_2 (partial pressure of oxygen [O_2] in arterial blood), but would not correct the carbon dioxide deficit.
b. Restraint is likely to increase the client's anxiety and worsen the hysteria, which might increase the respiratory rate, further lowering the $PaCO_2$.
d. The most likely problem is respiratory alkalosis due to hyperventilation. Drinking an electrolyte solution would not correct that problem. If breathing into a paper bag does not rapidly relieve the symptoms, other causes should be considered.

9. **Correct answer is b.** Dextran interferes with blood coagulation, thereby increasing the risk for bleeding.

a. Hyperkalemia occurs when stored blood is administered. Dextran is not a blood product, so it does not cause that problem.

c. Alkalosis can result from metabolism of citrate used to preserve stored blood. Dextran does not contain citrate, so alkalosis is not a problem with dextran.
d. Fluid overload is more likely. Dextran expands plasma volume by increasing the osmotic pressure. This client should be monitored for fluid retention.

10. **Correct answer is a.** Nutritional recovery syndrome is caused by hypophosphatemia related to influx of phosphorus into cells as anabolism occurs. Muscle weakness is an important sign that can be detected by testing the client's grip strength.

b. Deep-tendon reflexes become hyperactive in hypomagnesemia.
c. Carpal spasms (Trousseau's sign) indicate tetany—a sign of hypocalcemia.
d. Hypoactive bowel sounds indicate decreased bowel motility—a sign of hypokalemia.

11. **Correct answer is c.** Oral fluid replacement is preferred if the child is able to drink and not developing hypovolemic shock. Water and electrolytes should be replaced, and glucose is used because it facilitates absorption of sodium in the small intestine and provides kcal.

a. The use of water without electrolytes can lead to dilutional hyponatremia.
b and **d.** IV fluids would be used if the child is unable to drink or has signs of impending hypovolemic shock. In this case, parenteral therapy should not be necessary.

12. **Correct answer is b.** The elderly have reduced lung elasticity, diminished alveolar ventilation, and accumulation of bronchial secretions, all of which contribute to CO_2 retention. An elevated $PaCO_2$ can cause acidosis. To help this client eliminate more CO_2, the nurse should teach breathing exercises with a prolonged expiratory phase.

a. Drinking acidic juices does not increase the risk of acidosis. Fluid intake should be encouraged to promote adequate renal function so that the client excretes hydrogen ions adequately and reduces the risk for metabolic acidosis.

c. Improving potassium intake does not reduce the risk of acidosis. CO_2 retention and impaired hydrogen ion excretion are the causes of risk for acidosis that need to be addressed.

d. This would prevent acid reflux if the client had a hiatal hernia. It does not address the causes of acidosis.

13. **Correct answer is d.** Tachypnea may reflect hyperventilation in an effort to blow off CO_2. This suggests metabolic acidosis due to accumulation of lactic acid as cells break down. The physician should be notified so that ABGs can be checked and treatment initiated.

a. A slight temperature elevation due to fluid loss is common after trauma.

b. The systolic pressure often falls after trauma. A narrowing pulse pressure is an early sign of hypovolemic shock. A pulse pressure lower than 20 should be reported. This client's pulse pressure is 38.

c. A pulse rate greater than 120 suggests shock and should be reported.

14. **Correct answer is b.** The injury places this client at risk for central diabetes insipidus secondary to damage to the pituitary. Deficient ADH results in production of very dilute urine. If water is not replaced adequately, hypernatremia will develop.

a. Head injuries can cause syndrome of inappropriate ADH, with fluid volume excess. This client's polyuria and low specific gravity indicate a deficit of ADH.

c. Deficient aldosterone release would reflect an adrenal problem. Polyuria usually produces hypokalemia.

d. Increased intracranial pressure, which is expected with head injury, does not produce abnormal temperatures during the

compensatory phase. Abnormal hypothalamic function during the decompensatory phase results in hyperthermia.

15. **Correct answer is d.** Hypokalemia is one cause of adynamic ileus. Steroid use promotes potassium loss.

a and b. Urine and serum osmolality are helpful in evaluation of fluid balance. This client's hypovolemia is due to third spacing of fluid in the intestine. It is not the cause of the adynamic ileus.

c. Arterial blood gases are used to identify acid-base imbalances. Adynamic ileus is not usually caused by acid-base imbalance.

16. **Correct answer is a.** The client with pancreatitis may develop any acid-base imbalance. The nurse must consider the client's clinical condition to determine which imbalance a specific client is at risk for. Because this client has both ascites and pleural effusion, lung expansion is restricted. Narcotics cause hypoventilation. CO_2 retention with respiratory acidosis is most likely.

b. Pain can stimulate hyperventilation and produce respiratory alkalosis. This client's pain is controlled, so respiratory alkalosis is not likely.

c. Renal failure due to hypovolemia would put this client at risk for metabolic acidosis. Renal function is not impaired in this case.

d. Gastric fluid losses through vomiting or gastric suction would produce metabolic alkalosis. Neither of these is occurring in this client.

17. **Correct answer is a.** The client needs increased intake of potassium. Lasix increases potassium excretion, and hypokalemia predisposes clients to digitalis toxicity. Many fruits are good sources of potassium.

b. Turkey is high in phosphorus and chloride. Poultry is not a good source of potassium.

c and **d.** Breads and dairy products are high in sodium and need to be limited by clients with congestive heart failure.

18. **Correct answer is a.** Decreased pH indicates acidosis. The client shows signs of airway obstruction and air trapping, which would elevate $PaCO_2$ and produce respiratory acidosis.

    b. A low $PaCO_2$ would occur with hyperventilation. The client is at risk for CO_2 retention, which would produce a $PaCO_2$ greater than 45.
    c. This is a normal bicarbonate level. It is not indicative of any acid-base imbalance. Altered bicarbonate levels cause metabolic acidosis or alkalosis. The client is at risk for respiratory acidosis.
    d. This is within the normal range for base excess. In respiratory acidosis, the base excess becomes positive as the kidneys compensate.

19. **Correct answer is c.** Serum potassium of 2.6 mEq/L indicates severe—even life-threatening—hypokalemia, which must be corrected as quickly as is safely possible. Carefully paced IV administration of appropriately diluted potassium solution is indicated, with constant monitoring for cardiac changes by electrocardiogram.

    a and **b.** Neither dietary potassium nor oral potassium supplements would correct the hypokalemia quickly enough to minimize the possibility of dangerous cardiac arrhythmias.
    d. Adding potassium to the dialysate used for peritoneal dialysis would prevent further loss of potassium and would increase the serum potassium level only slowly. This clinical situation requires more rapid correction than the peritoneal dialysis route would provide.

20. **Correct answer is a.** NSAIDs cause sodium and fluid retention. They can also cause renal damage, which could speed progression to end-stage renal disease.

b. Beta-adrenergic antagonists s‎ avoided, because they may reduce perfusion. Adrenergic agonists are contraindicated.
c. Loop diuretics may be used to im‎ urine output. Loss of electrolytes due‎ uretic use can be beneficial when ele‎ levels are high.
d. As kidney function decreases, eryth‎ poietin, which stimulates red blood cell duction, is decreased. Iron and B vitami‎ may reduce the anemia that results.

21. **Correct answer is b.** PTH raises serum calcium levels by shifting calcium from bones into serum. Ectopic PTH secretion in creases the risk for hypercalcemia.

    a. PTH does not alter metabolism as thyroid hormones do. PTH regulates calcium balance.
    c. Ectopic secretion of ACTH would produce hypokalemia.
    d. Ectopic ADH production causes syndrome of inappropriate ADH. PTH does not alter ADH production.

22. **Correct answer is b.** High-dose Cytoxan induces dilutional hyponatremia due to increased ADH secretion. Headache can be a sign of developing cerebral edema, which indicates water intoxication. Many of the signs of hyponatremia are difficult for a client to monitor at home or are indistinguishable from the side effects of chemotherapy. Headache is an early sign the client can recognize.

    a. Peripheral edema occurs with extracellular fluid excess, not with intracellular fluid excess. In intracellular fluid excess due to hyponatremia, fluid is retained inside cells.
    c. Thirst is a sign of hypernatremia, not hyponatremia. High-dose Cytoxan causes hyponatremia.
    d. Leg cramps are associated with deficits of potassium and calcium. Cytoxan is most likely to cause hyponatremia.

is c. Acidosis causes in-
_____ idosis is corrected, in-
_____ effective and the risk of
_____ ases. Hypoglycemia
_____ sweating.

_____ skin occurs with fluid vol-
_____ ketosis. With treatment,
_____ moisture would return to

_____ ul breathing occurs in severe
_____ acidosis, as the lungs compensate
_____ ng off CO_2. As acidosis is corrected,
_____ tions return to normal.

_____ arrhea may occur with elevated potas-
_____ During treatment, hypokalemia,
_____ ch slows peristalsis, is more likely.

24. **Correct answer is d.** Thrombosis is a
common complication of HHNK coma, due to
decreased tissue perfusion and increased
blood viscosity. Leg exercises decrease venous stasis, thereby reducing the risk.

a. The client will have a severe fluid volume deficit. The head should be kept lower
to promote cerebral perfusion.
b. This would be appropriate if the client
were semicomatose. Oral fluids are encouraged if the client can drink.
c. This would be appropriate for a client
with chronic obstructive pulmonary disease,
because metabolism of carbohydrate produces more CO_2 than fat metabolism does.
Leg exercises are not helpful in HHNK
coma.